Low Fiber Low Residue Diet

A 2-Phase Plan for Flares and Recovery (With Food Lists, Reintroduction Steps, Meal Plans and Easy Recipes)

mf

Disclaimer

This guide is provided for informational and educational purposes only and should not be interpreted as medical, nutritional, or professional advice. The author is not a licensed physician, nurse, dietitian, or mental health provider. Reading this guide does not establish a patient-provider relationship of any kind.

Always seek the guidance of a qualified healthcare professional before starting, changing, or discontinuing any supplement, diet, or lifestyle program. If you are pregnant, breastfeeding, managing a chronic medical condition, or taking prescription medications, consult your physician or pharmacist before considering any product mentioned in this guide.

The author and publisher make no representations or warranties regarding accuracy, applicability, fitness, or completeness of the information contained herein. While every effort has been made to ensure scientific accuracy and currency, medical knowledge and research evolve continually. Readers are responsible for verifying information and making decisions in consultation with licensed professionals.

Use of this guide and any information contained within it is at your own risk. The author and publisher disclaim all liability for any loss, injury, or adverse outcome that may result from the use or misuse of this material.

Table of Contents

Introduction

If you have just received a diagnosis that requires a low fiber or low residue diet, you may already know how daily life can be disrupted by digestive problems. Abdominal pain, unpredictable bowel movements, ongoing bloating, and food fear are constant challenges during digestive flares, after gastrointestinal surgery, or while managing conditions like strictures and slow transit constipation.

Every meal can become a source of anxiety, as foods that were once safe may now trigger discomfort or more severe symptoms. For many adults, these struggles are not just physical. The loss of control over your diet and worrying about what will happen if symptoms spiral out of control can quickly erode your confidence in everyday life.

Failing to manage these symptoms well carries clear consequences. When flare symptoms remain unchecked, you may face urgent hospital visits, a slower recovery from surgery, or even blockages of the bowel that threaten overall health. Eating the wrong foods can cause new pain, swelling, or even lead to dangerous complications that delay healing.

There is also the risk of nutritional gaps from cutting out whole food groups, especially when avoiding whole grains, raw fruits and vegetables, beans, and most dairy for long stretches. These trade-offs cause more than inconvenience; they affect your healing, energy, and mood.

This guide will give you practical skills to regain your footing. First, it helps build targeted symptom control so you can weather flares or rough periods with safer meal choices and less guesswork. With clear steps, you will learn how to gradually reintroduce foods as symptoms settle, using a stepwise system so you do not go too quickly or too slowly.

Planning meals that work with your restrictions will become more manageable, and you will gain the tools to spot hidden nutritional risks before they become problems. Along with suggested menus and adaptable food lists, you will develop greater confidence in every food decision you make.

Every guide has edges, and this one is no exception. Here, you will not find recommendations for children, diets targeting illnesses outside the gut, or advice for long-term high-fiber eating. Urgent or complicated medical emergencies also require care outside the scope of this book, such as in-hospital management or specialist consultation. The instructions and tools here are designed for typical adult experiences with digestive disorders or surgery, where home-based dietary changes are both needed and safe.

In this guide, you will:

- Unpack how fiber and residue actually work in the digestive system, and why reducing them can calm symptoms.
- Learn clinical guidelines that define when to tighten restrictions, when to expand, and how long to stay at each stage.

- Follow step-by-step frameworks to help make practical food choices at any phase of your journey, with support to modify meals based on your personal response.
- Use flexible models for stocking your kitchen, prepping meals, and changing eating habits without feeling deprived.
- Apply simple cooking techniques that improve food tolerance and minimize digestive stress.
- Use troubleshooting tips to get ahead of common setbacks like unintentional fiber intake, new symptoms, or boredom with repetitive meals.
- Build a personalized plan for reintroducing foods, supported by sustainable strategies for long-term recovery.

Through careful explanation, real-world examples, and easy-to-use frameworks, this guide is your companion for not only surviving tough digestive phases, but also reclaiming day-to-day control, one meal at a time. Always consult your healthcare provider for guidance that fits your unique needs.

Fundamentals of Fiber, Residue, and the Digestive System

What happens at the intersection of food and the digestive tract can shape how you feel each day. To understand a low fiber or low residue diet, you first need to know how different foods interact at every stage of digestion. This chapter demystifies the roles of fiber and residue, examining how each contributes to digestion, stool formation, and the burden on the gut. Through several practical comparisons and detailed explanations, you will see why certain foods feel rougher on your system, and how smart food choices can help you feel better.

Start by picturing your digestive system as a carefully tuned conveyor belt. What you put on it—soluble or insoluble fiber, residue-prone foods, refined grains, or processed options—can speed up, slow down, or even jam the belt. Each type of component acts differently, and knowing these differences is crucial for clearer decision making when you adjust your diet for symptom relief or recovery.

Fiber and residue spectrum: a comparison

To clarify confusion, compare fiber and residue as two related but different kinds of leftovers in the digestive process. Both influence stool, but they arise from different food sources, play separate roles in digestion, and vary in how the body processes them.

If you sort common foods along a spectrum, you quickly notice these distinctions:

Component	Source Examples	Main Role in Digestion	Digestibility	Effect on Stool Formation
Soluble Fiber	Oats, barley, apples (no peel), beans (if allowed)	Slows digestion, forms gel	Partially digested	Softer, bulkier stools
Insoluble Fiber	Wheat bran, raw veggies, whole grains	Adds bulk, speeds movement	Not digested	Larger, harder stools
Non-fiber Residue	Lactose in milk, undigested chunks of protein, tough connective tissue in meats, additives	Minimal digestive role, may ferment or pass through	Often not digested	Increased stool volume or gas
Low-Residue Foods	White bread, white rice, peeled canned fruits	Gentlest transit, minimizes gut work	Mostly digested	Lower stool volume, less frequency

Soluble fiber, typically found in the inner part of grains and the flesh of some fruits and vegetables, forms a gel when mixed with water. This slows stomach emptying and helps soften stool. Insoluble fiber the tough outer husk of grains, skins, and raw plant structures scours the bowel, adding bulk and promoting regular movement.

Residue sweeps up whatever is left undigested, from milk sugars in those who lack the proper enzymes, to connective tissues in certain cuts of meat, and additives that slip past the body's natural grinders.

Foods lowest in both fiber and residue pass smoothly through, producing little undigested matter. These include options made from highly refined flour (think white bread and pasta), soft well-cooked vegetables with no skins or seeds, lean tender meats, and small measured servings of certain dairy if tolerated. They help reduce the workload for the gut, an advantage during flares or after surgery when your system needs the least resistance.

How soluble and insoluble fiber show themselves in real foods

When you walk through a supermarket, you see the choices lined up: a loaf of dense whole-wheat bread, a shiny red apple, a bowl of oatmeal, a bag of white rice. To build a gentler diet, you need to spot the working parts soluble and insoluble fiber and understand how each behaves once eaten.

Soluble fiber is the portion that dissolves in liquid, forming a sticky gel. Oatmeal is a classic example. When cooked, it becomes smooth and thick; the body partially digests it, resulting in a softer, sometimes bulkier stool. Ripe bananas also offer soluble fiber, making them a gentler option during mild symptoms. Meanwhile, lentils though soft when cooked are rich in this kind of fiber as well as insoluble types, which excludes them from most low-residue plans.

Insoluble fiber is what gives leafy greens their structure or forms the grainy skin on an apple. Whole-wheat bread is loaded with it. Eat a salad of raw spinach or chew on a bran muffin, and your gut receives a non-digestible roughness. If you are healthy, this can keep things moving along. But for those in digestive distress, insoluble fiber quickly becomes the enemy—it bulks up stool, increases mechanical strain, and often leads to pain, gas, and urgent trips to the bathroom.

To see this in action, look at two breakfast bowls:

- **Bowl A:** Cream of wheat (refined, almost no fiber), topped with strained canned peach slices.
- **Bowl B:** Bran flakes, raw apple slices (with skin), a sprinkle of walnuts.

Bowl A sits light and mostly digests, producing little residue and a softer, smaller stool load. Bowl B, ideal for those with no GI risk, delivers a large, bulky stool that strains an injured or inflamed bowel. The first is safe during strict restriction phases; the second waits until symptoms completely ease.

Residue arises from more than fiber: main contributors to undigested bulk

Residue is best thought of as what remains after digestion—not just undigested fiber, but remnants from many sources. It appears as the sum of fiber, undigested proteins, certain carbohydrates, and even food additives that resist breakdown.

Think of the process this way:

1. You chew and swallow food.
2. The stomach and intestines extract usable nutrients and water.
3. Soluble fibers are partially broken down, yielding a soft gel that slows absorption.
4. Insoluble fibers, dairy in some people, and unabsorbed fats, proteins, or additives pass through, contributing to stool mass.
5. The colon gathers this remaining material fiber fragments, tough meat, undigested milk sugars, and additives into stool, along with water and a bit of mucus.
6. The result leaves the body as a formed stool, which may sometimes be bulky.

Among the key contributors:

- **Insoluble fibers:** rampant in whole grains, bran, and tough vegetables. These are not digested.
- **Soluble fibers:** partially digested, but some remains as gel-like residue.
- **Lactose: f**or many adults who lack enough lactase enzyme, milk products leave behind sugars that create gas and soft, heavy stool.
- **Tough proteins and meat fibers:** gristly, heavily marbled cuts tend to be poorly digested, leaving fragments.
- **Additives:** artificial sweeteners like sorbitol or gums in processed foods often resist digestion.

Eating low-residue usually focuses on limiting all these sources. Not only are whole foods like beans, seeds, and raw veggies out, but also tough and fatty meats or more than modest amounts of milk.

Each source adds to your digestive work, making symptoms worse when your gut is vulnerable.

If you want less residue, focus on these strategies:

- Use white rice and plain pasta instead of brown rice or whole grain noodles.
- Peel fruits and vegetables, then cook them well. Soft, skinless, seedless produce is safest.
- Select lean, tender meats and avoid tough cuts.
- Limit milk intake to no more than two cups daily, unless your provider says to avoid it completely or allows lactose-free substitutes.
- Steer clear of nuts, seeds, dried fruit, popcorn, and anything with whole-wheat, bran, or coconut.

What happens to stool and gut workload when fiber and residue are reduced

People often wonder what real changes occur after shifting to a low fiber, low residue diet. Health professionals use this approach carefully, aiming for less bowel movement frequency, lower stool volume, and decreased pain or risk of blockages during sensitive periods.

Consider the gut before the change:

- Stool volume is large, frequent, sometimes urgent.
- Consistency is bulkier and can be hard to pass for those with strictures or slow transit.
- Symptoms such as pain, gas, cramping, or bloating are common.

- The gut must push undigested matter along, straining inflamed or healing tissue.

Now, after shifting to low-residue choices:

- Stool becomes smaller and less frequent. For some, this feels like relief; for others, it gives the bowel a rest during recovery or flare-ups.
- The effort needed to move food along decreases, which is crucial for avoiding further trauma.
- The risk of new flare-ups, blockages, or surgical complications lowers because the gut faces less stress and irritation.

For example, a patient recovering from bowel surgery should avoid high-residue foods such as raw carrot sticks and whole oats, since these force the gut to squeeze and churn when gentleness is needed. Substituting with white toast, well-cooked peeled potatoes, and clear juice reduces mechanical strain and gives the healing tissue a much-needed break. As a result, pain and gas decrease, and stool passes more easily with less bulk.

This approach works for those with inflammatory conditions too. Crohn's disease or ulcerative colitis comes with raw, inflamed sections of bowel that dislike abrasion. Keeping residue down can limit symptom intensity and speed the pathway to recovery.

However, reducing residue is not without trade-offs. When you cut back too long or without supervision, nutritional gaps develop. The same process that minimizes gut stress can limit intake of vitamins, minerals, and healthy plant compounds. Any period over two weeks should include a multivitamin and regular check-ins with your provider.

Checkpoints for safe, effective diet decisions

When considering any shift in your diet whether tightening restrictions or navigating the next step in recovery use these anatomical and metabolic checkpoints as repeat reference points. **They help ensure changes support both immediate comfort and long-term health:**

1. **Mouth and esophagus:** Are foods soft and easy to swallow? Avoid chunks that can strain chewing or passage.
2. **Stomach:** Does the meal feel light or heavy? Meals overloaded with fat, tough meat, or coarse grains sit longer and may worsen discomfort.
3. **Small intestine:** Are there elements that will be too rough, such as whole beans, seeds, or bran? Aim for gentle choices during vulnerable times.
4. **Colon:** Is stool passing easily, without pain, urgency, or bloating? Softer, smaller stools mean your regimen is likely working.
5. **Metabolic balance:** Are you getting at least some protein, enough fluids, and basic micronutrients? If not, add a daily multivitamin and consult a professional for modifications.
6. **Monitoring symptoms:** If symptoms worsen, or new ones appear especially pain, fever, or persistent vomiting, pause and ask your provider for direction before making further adjustments.

You can use the following reference as a mental guide card:

- Are today's foods low in fiber, skins, seeds, and tough proteins?
- Have all fruits or vegetables been peeled, cooked, and de-seeded?
- Is milk intake within permitted levels, or replaced if intolerant?
- Is stool becoming easier, smaller, and less frequent—without new symptoms?
- Have supplement needs, especially a daily multivitamin, been addressed if restrictions last longer than two weeks?
- Have you checked with a healthcare professional before extending or expanding the diet?

Each meal offers a chance to protect healing tissue, reduce pain, and control symptoms. Using these checkpoints keeps your diet in harmony with your anatomy and helps avoid nutritional roadblocks.

Mastering the fundamentals of fiber and residue unlocks more confident management of your digestive health. Soluble and insoluble fiber differ not just in chemistry, but in how they interact with the body and affect stool. Non-fiber residue compounds the process, making food selection a careful balancing act between comfort and completeness.

Lowering both fiber and residue relieves everyday strain on the gut, leading to smaller, less disruptive stools and fewer symptoms when it matters most. At each step, the checkpoints above serve as guideposts ensuring that phase transitions and food choices build toward healing, not setback.

As you move forward in this guide, you will build on these core ideas. Knowing specifically which foods to limit, how and when to expand your options, and how to monitor symptoms through every stage will give you the structure and confidence needed for full recovery and safe, sustainable choices.

Keep this foundation in mind whenever your symptoms shift or new decisions arise. By staying grounded in how food interacts with your digestive system at every level, you can approach meal planning as an active part of your healing and not just a series of tough restrictions.

Clinical Indications and Contraindications for Diet Use

A quick question often brings clarity: "Who should follow a low fiber or low residue diet?" To explore this, let's start with the reasons someone might need to use this plan, sorted by how quickly the diet needs to start, how long it's used, and key clinical features.

Rapid response is sometimes required. Certain digestive scenarios demand swift restriction of rough, bulky foods. Others call for short-term gentle eating during recovery, while some conditions benefit from precautionary use for a few days. Each situation differs in urgency and expected diet length.

Conditions Are Not Equal: Sorting by Clinical Urgency

Acute cases where quick action is needed include bowel obstruction or strictures. These block passage, making immediate reduction of fiber and residue critical to prevent pain, further blockage, or surgical complications. Diet restriction usually starts as soon as symptoms appear or as advised following imaging and examination by healthcare staff. Duration is shortest here, often only until the blockage passes or can be safely managed, which can be a matter of days to a couple of weeks.

Post-surgery patients form the next group. After operations on the bowel, the gut must heal. In these cases, doctors often prescribe a low fiber, low residue diet to reduce mechanical strain and give tissue time to recover. This phase usually runs until healing progresses enough for a gradual return to normal eating. For some, this takes a few days; for others, a few weeks, depending on the operation and recovery speed.

Inflammatory bowel disease (such as Crohn's disease or ulcerative colitis) flares make up another category. During acute flares, digestive tissue becomes inflamed and sensitive. The diet is used to avoid worsening symptoms such as diarrhea, cramping, and gas. Here, restriction usually starts with a flare and continues until symptoms settle, after which a gradual re-introduction begins.

Some people deal with long-term slow transit constipation or functional difficulties. The diet may be recommended for limited stretches to break a cycle of pain or difficulty passing stool, but only with close supervision.

Chronic use is very rarely recommended. Long-term complete restriction can cause nutritional deficiencies or worsen overall health. The most typical pattern is for temporary use, unless an individual's anatomy or repeated complications absolutely require it.

Visual Key for Duration:

- **Acute (days):** Obstruction, severe strictures, surgery
- **Intermediate (1–2 weeks):** Flare recovery, post-illness healing
- **Transitional (>2 weeks, caution):** Only under strict provider guidance

Quick Reference: Where Use Is Safe, Where It Carries Risks

Matching the right diet to the right scenario calls for a clear balance sheet. The following table summarizes main uses where the approach is helpful, versus where sticking with it too long may tip into harm.

Therapeutic Use / Duration	Key Benefit	Risk of Prolonged Restriction
Acute Obstruction, Stricture	Rapid symptom relief, prevents further blockage; reduces risk during healing	Missed nutrients after >2 weeks; muscle loss; worsening weakness
Post-bowel Surgery	Lowers gut strain for healing tissues; supports smoother recovery	Protein and micronutrient gaps if extended beyond advice
IBD Flare	Reduces pain, diarrhea, urgency for easier recovery; minimizes gut irritation	Reduced intake of fiber, vitamins, and minerals—especially plant nutrients—if continued longer than needed
Slow Transit Constipation, Gastroparesis (very limited use)	Rest for slowed gut; test if symptoms improve, short span only	Constipation can worsen, nutritional problems may arise
Patient preference, mild digestive distress (rare)	Used to trial symptom changes or during NPO transitions	Delayed identification of other causes, missed diagnosis

In each of these situations, the main goal is to shield a vulnerable digestive system without blocking the intake of vital nutrients for longer than necessary. If the reason for eating this way disappears, or if symptoms resolve, quick transition back to a less restricting diet is best. Lingering on the restricted diet leads to the body missing out on plant nutrients, vitamins, and minerals that only come from a more varied menu.

Clinical Scenarios: When to Use and When Not to

A low residue diet is recommended in specific situations where reducing stool bulk and easing gastrointestinal activity are important. Appropriate indications include acute bowel obstruction, recent bowel surgery, or active inflammatory bowel disease (IBD) flare. During these times, limiting fiber and residue can help minimize symptoms and support healing. As symptoms resolve or healing progresses, dietary fiber is gradually reintroduced under medical supervision.

It is important to avoid starting a low residue diet without a clear clinical indication. Using this diet for general wellness, weight loss, or as a fad can be unnecessarily restrictive and potentially harmful, leading to inadequate nutrition and masking important symptoms. Chronic use without medical need may delay appropriate diagnosis and treatment.

The diet should be discontinued when symptoms improve, healing is confirmed, or if no benefit is observed after a reasonable trial. New or worsening symptoms such as weakness, unintended weight loss, or constipation should prompt reevaluation and discontinuation of the diet.

Understanding these evidence-based indications helps ensure the low residue diet is used safely and effectively, minimizing risks to overall health.

Key Questions to Ask Before a Provider Visit

When preparing to talk with your healthcare provider about starting, continuing, or ending a low fiber or low residue diet, readiness begins with specific information. Providers need a full, clear account of what is happening past, present, and as symptoms evolve.

Bring answers to these questions:

- What specific symptoms started, and when? (Example: sharp pain, diarrhea, unplanned weight loss, bloating)
- Were there any clear triggers? (Change in diet, medication, recent activity, stress)
- Are there warning signs suggestive of "red flag" conditions? (Fevers, bleeding, severe pain not responding to simple plans, vomiting that will not stop, sudden loss of appetite)
- Did you notice escalation—worsening pattern, new symptoms, or decline despite dietary change?
- How long have you been following low fiber, and what foods have you included or avoided? Are you taking a multivitamin with minerals if more than two weeks have passed on the diet?
- Have you checked for lactose intolerance, and used lactose-free dairy or none at all if necessary?
- Are bowel movements easier, less frequent, or maybe even too infrequent?
- What supportive measures have you tried (hydration, gentle exercise, medication changes)?

Arriving prepared with these details allows the provider to quickly decide if you are a good candidate for continuing the plan, need adjustments, or should change strategy altogether. Accurate, honest answers help catch any brewing problems before they become serious.

Signals That the Diet Is Failing or Has Gone On Too Long

Sometimes, despite best intentions, the plan does not work as hoped. Other times, lingering on low fiber or low residue foods crosses into causing harm. Recognizing signs of overuse or failed benefit ensures safe, effective care.

Failure looks like:

- New or worsening symptoms after starting the diet (more pain, new constipation, muscle weakness, fatigue)
- No improvement in stool frequency or consistency after several days, even when following the recommendations closely
- Signs of nutritional gaps (hair loss, skin changes, mouth sores, unexpected weight changes, repeated infections)
- Lowered energy, trouble focusing, or muscle loss
- Signs of dehydration or electrolyte imbalance (dizziness, shaking, palpitations)

If these appear, prompt steps are needed:

1. Contact your provider to discuss symptoms and next steps.
2. Ask for review of supplements if on the diet longer than two weeks; ensure a multivitamin with minerals is included.
3. If you are lactose intolerant, ensure all dairy intake is completely restricted or lactose-free products are substituted.

4. Consider advancing fiber slowly under guidance if original symptoms (e.g., cramping, diarrhea) have resolved, to lower the risk of long-term problems.
5. Monitor closely. Keep track of symptoms and review them with your healthcare team often.
6. Adjust hydration and seek help for persistent constipation, which sometimes occurs if fiber is cut too far.

Remember, this diet works best as a short-term intervention, not a permanent way of eating. It helps your gut recover or manage short-term symptoms, but it does not provide the nutrients needed for lifelong health. A key sign of responsible use is planning for reintroduction and regular review with your provider.

Practical Details: Foods to Focus On, Foods to Avoid

The choices you make each day on this diet should reflect both your current health needs and guidance from your health team. Refined grains, skinless fruits and soft cooked vegetables, lean well-cooked meats, and lactose-limited dairy make up the backbone of each meal. Foods to skip include whole grains, raw vegetables, seeds, nuts, dried fruit, tough meat, coconut, popcorn, and most unstrained juices.

Keys to a Successful Dietary Transition

Moving off this plan is safer and smoother with a gradual approach. Once the reason for restriction has passed healing completes, a flare calms, a blockage clears and begins increasing fiber a little at a time. Start with soft, cooked, peeled fruits or vegetables, and slowly add back higher fiber items, always drinking plenty of fluids. Record any symptom changes as you go.

If you notice any trouble, return of pain, bloating, change in stool, adjust the speed of reintroduction or seek advice. Most people experience better results when fiber comes back in phases, not all at once.

Nutrition Safeguards During Restriction

While following a low fiber or low residue plan, nutritional gaps can sneak in if care is not taken. Risks grow higher after two weeks, especially for vitamins, minerals, and adequate protein. Counter this by:

- Taking a daily multivitamin and mineral supplement.
- Checking with your provider before using nutrition drinks or powders, to confirm they fit your phase.
- Eating a variety of allowed foods: refined grains, soft cooked fruits and vegetables (peeled, de-seeded), lean meats, lactose-free dairy if appropriate, eggs, and clear juices.

Pay attention to protein intake, especially during recovery phases. Loss of appetite is common, but insufficient protein slows healing. Seek advice if you cannot meet your needs with the foods allowed.

Maintaining a Communication Loop

Perhaps the most effective way to remain safe is to maintain regular discussion with your healthcare providers. Advance planning, symptom diaries, and clear reports of any changes support better care and faster solutions. If your symptoms recur, or you feel uncertain about your progress, reach out before making major diet changes.

If any recommendation in this chapter causes confusion, do not hesitate to ask for clarification. Healthcare providers are there to guide, troubleshoot, and adjust plans to your needs.

Avoiding Common Pitfalls

Some traps can derail your progress:

- Avoid ignoring early signs that the diet is no longer helping or is beginning to cause harm (fatigue, nutritional changes, or bowel movement changes).
- Do not guess about safe reintroduction timelines—let your healthcare team outline the pace, especially after surgery or major flares.
- Be honest about any difficulties following the plan, including cost, meal monotony, or gaps in protein.

Quick Correction Steps

Spotting mistakes or over-extension early prevents more serious issues. Actions include:

- Gradually reintroduce peeled, cooked fruits and vegetables first when symptoms resolve or your provider advises.
- Revisit your supplement routine if on the plan for more than two weeks; adjust as advised.
- Watch hydration and fiber carefully, especially if constipation develops as you add foods back.
- For persistent unexplained symptoms, return to your healthcare team for a targeted workup rather than self-adjust.

A low fiber or low residue diet is a targeted approach for specific digestive problems. When used in the right scenario and for the correct duration, it brings acute relief, reduces mechanical strain, and gives the bowel a break when it needs it most. However, overuse or misapplied restrictions can introduce new risks. Success relies on recognizing when to start, how long to continue, and when to stop. Frequent, open communication with your provider, careful symptom monitoring, and a staged return to broader eating top the list of best practices.

With this understanding, you will be ready to use the plan wisely protecting healing tissue and controlling symptoms without falling into the trap of excessive restriction or delayed recovery.

The Two-Phase System for Flare Management and Recovery

Managing a digestive flare or recovering after bowel surgery is often a process of steps and transitions, rather than a quick fix. The two-phase system for flare management and recovery offers a structured approach to achieve relief, encourage healing, and safely move back to a regular eating pattern. This chapter walks through the logic and sequence of the two-phase system, using practical instructions, clear rules, and real examples to help you apply it with confidence.

The two-phase system splits your journey into a short, strict period Phase 1 where meals are tailored to quiet symptoms, followed by a gradual recovery Phase 2 that reintroduces variety and nutrients as your gut calms down. Knowing when and how to make each transition is the key to balancing relief and full recovery.

Phase 1 and Phase 2: Summary Roadmap

At the start of a digestive flare, bowel obstruction, or after bowel surgery, your provider may guide you into Phase 1. This phase means following a low fiber, low residue diet as strictly as possible. The purpose is to minimize the amount of undigested material passing through your system, which can reduce symptoms such as diarrhea, gas, cramping, and pain. Foods tend to be basic: refined white breads, white rice, soft cooked or canned fruits and vegetables (without skins or seeds), well-cooked lean meats, eggs, and lactose-limited dairy.

The timeline for Phase 1 varies. For some, the acute phase may last only a few days such as after a colonoscopy or brief post-surgical period. For others, especially during severe inflammatory flares, it may take up to two weeks to see symptoms quiet down enough to step forward. It is rare to stay in this phase longer than two weeks. Doing so can create risks for hunger, nutrient gaps, muscle loss, or even increased constipation.

Once symptoms have settled, and your provider clears you, Phase 2 begins. In this stage, fiber and residue-causing foods are reintroduced very slowly, always monitoring for any sign of returning symptoms. This is often called the recovery or ramp-up phase. Each step adds back more variety—perhaps starting with one new fruit, one more vegetable, or a small portion of whole grain at a time, and waiting at least a day or two before making another change. The end goal is to reach a full, balanced diet, as tolerated.

Gateposts for moving between phases include both clear symptom milestones and time-based checks. For example, you may be allowed to exit Phase 1 once you have had two or three days with solid improvement—less pain, formed stools, no severe bloating—and basic lab work or medical exams support safe progress. Phase 2 can last from several days to a few weeks, with the pace determined by your body's reaction and continued guidance from your medical team.

Symptom Stabilization: When to Start and End Each Phase

Recognizing stability is easier with a set of real signals. Common complaints that call for starting Phase 1 include persistent diarrhea, sharp or crampy abdominal pain, bloating, or recent bowel surgery. If you are experiencing these, your health provider may suggest immediately switching to a low residue pattern to let the gut rest.

For clarity, here are examples of symptoms that flag readiness to begin Phase 1:

- Four or more bowel movements per day, loose or watery in texture
- Abdominal pain that stays level or worsens with usual meals
- Visible abdominal swelling, not explained by weight gain
- Nausea, mild vomiting, or loss of appetite after solid foods
- Recent intestinal surgery with orders to “start light and progress slowly”

Once in Phase 1, your daily routine focuses on gentle eating, tracking changes, and limiting intake to safe foods. It is helpful to write down what you eat and how you feel.

Clear signs to exit Phase 1 and begin Phase 2 include:

- Stool pattern has normalized or nearly so (formed, less frequent)
- Pain and bloating have greatly decreased or resolved
- No new or worsening symptoms for at least 48 hours
- Appetite starts to return
- Any fever, severe pain, or vomiting has fully resolved

It is not necessary to wait for total "normalcy," just for symptoms to improve enough that your gut seems ready for more. If symptoms worsen with reintroduction, step back to the previous safe set of foods for a few days, then try again.

Benefits–Risks Weighing: What Each Phase Brings

Short-term use of a low fiber, low residue diet can rapidly ease many digestive symptoms. These include less diarrhea, lower abdominal discomfort, less gas, and less pressure on fresh surgical tissues. Choosing refined grains, soft proteins, and simple cooked produce means less bulk material travels through the colon, giving time for inflammation or surgical healing to settle.

The flip side of this relief is that such severe restriction can rob the body of nutrients in as little as two weeks. Fiber is removed, but so are vitamins, minerals, and plant compounds the body relies on. Constipation can become a problem, as can low energy, dry skin, sore mouth, or falling appetite. Protein may lag too, especially if meat, eggs, or dairy intake is cut for other reasons.

In each phase, benefits and risks play against each other.

Phase 1 Benefits:

- Fast reduction in pain, cramping, gas, and stool volume.
- Decreases risk of blockage or wound tension post-surgery.
- Small, easy-to-digest meals support a rest period for the gut.

Phase 1 Risks:

- If used for more than two weeks, there is a strong risk of low vitamin, mineral, and plant nutrient intake.
- Missed protein needs, slow healing, and even increased constipation.
- Loss of plant diversity that helps good bacteria thrive.

Phase 2 Benefits:

- Gradual fiber return may keep gut symptoms calm while improving overall well-being.
- Variety brings more taste, satisfaction, and wider nutrition.
- Protection against long-term nutritional gaps or loss of strength.

Phase 2 Risks:

- Too fast a reintroduction may bring symptoms back (bloating, pain, loose stools).
- Without careful tracking, food "triggers" may be overlooked.
- Some foods may not be tolerated at first, requiring careful selection and a slower pace.

The way to keep the advantages and dodge the hazards is to use the shortest needed course for Phase 1, start Phase 2 as soon as you can, and check in often with your provider about symptoms and progress. Supplements like a daily multivitamin may help if you need to stay restricted, but always ask first.

Transition Rules: When and How to Advance

Success with this two-phase system depends on knowing when your system is ready to move forward and having a clear way to track what happens at each step. **Providers often set basic rules for transition:**

1. Wait until key symptoms have stayed improved for at least two days.
2. If you have had no new pain, fever, or vomiting, and you are passing gas or stool without distress, prepare to increase variety.
3. Start Phase 2 by adding back one new food group or portion every 24–48 hours, unless you notice trouble.
4. Always keep a simple log—writing down what you tried, any symptoms, and your overall energy, digestion, and appetite.
5. Advance only as tolerated. Back up to a safe food set if problems appear.

Here is a practical sample log template you can copy into a notebook or digital file:

- Date: ________
- Meal(s): ____
- Foods added or changed: ____________________________
- Stool: # times, appearance ___________________________
- Symptoms today: (pain, bloat, N/V, appetite) _________
- Energy/mood/sleep: _________________________________
- Notes/next step: ____________________________________

Review this log each day and bring it to your next provider visit. It builds a clear story of your progress and flags patterns where foods or timing may connect to symptoms.

Day-in-the-Life Scenario: Meal Rhythm and Feedback

A typical day during strict flare management in Phase 1 is simple, repetitive, and focused on gentleness. Let's walk through a sample schedule. Assume sleep occurs from 10pm to 6am.

- **6:30 am: Wake up.** Drink a glass of clear juice (apple or grape), followed by a hot beverage such as decaf coffee with a splash of cream and sugar.
- **7:15 am: Breakfast.** Soft scrambled eggs, a slice of white toast with a bit of margarine and grape jelly (seedless), or a bowl of farina or cream of wheat. Hydrate with more juice or water.
- **10:00 am: Snack.** Small portion of soft, peeled canned fruit (peaches or pears in juice), a few saltine crackers.
- **12:30 pm: Lunch.** Baked chicken breast, white rice, canned carrots, maybe a small serving of green beans if tolerated. A soft dinner roll with a pat of margarine, or a plain hamburger on a white bun with ketchup and mayonnaise are also possibilities. Water, diluted juice, or decaf tea to drink.
- **3:00 pm: Snack.** Low-fat pudding or a small amount of American cheese (if dairy is tolerated), possibly a few plain crackers.
- **6:00 pm: Dinner.** Tender roast beef, white rice or mashed potatoes (without skins), cooked carrots or spinach, and a white dinner roll with butter. Could substitute broiled fish with a plain sauce and cooked green beans for variety.
- **8:30 pm: Gentle snack** if hungry, such as plain pasta with a dab of butter, or a fruit cocktail cup (no skins/seeds).

- **Bedtime: Herbal tea or water.** Note any symptoms such as and write them before sleeping.

  After each meal, pause to consider:

- Was there any change in pain, cramping, or bloating?
- Did the meal feel comfortable, or was there lingering fullness or nausea?
- Were bathroom trips normal, easier, or harder?
- Did your appetite stay steady, rise, or drop?

Recording these answers helps find the best pace for advancing your diet and quickly spots any setbacks.

In Phase 2, a day might look similar but feature gradual changes. One meal might include a small serving of well-cooked, skinless sweet potato, or a half portion of oatmeal instead of white toast.

Over a week, add back one fruit, one cooked vegetable, and increase the variety of lean meats or fish. The key is to try only one change at a time and give your system at least a full day to respond before introducing something new.

Closing the Loop: Adaptation, Reassessment, and Support

The two-phase system is not a locked sequence. Each person's progress is shaped by how symptoms improve, personal preferences, and any outside factors like medications, stress, or coexisting illnesses. Signs that you may need to slow down or temporarily return to stricter eating include swelling, unexpected pain, loose stools, or appetite loss.

Sustain success by:

- Keeping a simple food and symptom log during both phases.
- Reporting progress or problems to your healthcare provider, especially if planning to expand food choices.
- Taking supplements only as advised, especially if longer restriction is needed.
- Notice improvements and make adjustments as your gut recovers.

Some find emotional or practical value in partnering with a registered dietitian. This expert can review your food diary, spot hidden gaps, and help you fit the two-phase system into your wider lifestyle, preferences, and goals.

The two-phase system for flare management and recovery is designed to shield your digestive system in its most fragile states and then restore a satisfying, whole diet when the flare or injury passes. Used flexibly, with clear observations and steady dialogue with your care team, it brings symptom relief while reducing nutrition-related risks. Gradually adding foods back, instead of making sudden changes, helps improve your health for the long run.

By following this roadmap strict management when needed, attentive monitoring, and controlled expansion you can move through each stage safely, fueling recovery and building comfort with every meal. The ability to listen to your body, record your progress, and adapt as needed sets the foundation for both immediate relief and long-term health.

Food Lists and Gradual Ingredient Expansion

Building confidence in your food choices during a low fiber, low residue diet means knowing exactly what belongs on your plate at each step. Rather than relying on vague restrictions, you deserve a clear view: which foods unlock relief in the strict phase, which ones to test as you expand, and how to adapt choices to your own lifestyle. Bringing these foods together in an organized system lets you control symptoms, start broadening your menu when possible, and deal with common challenges, such as dietary preferences or food intolerances.

Approved and Restricted Foods for Each Phase

In the first, most restricted phase, selections are narrow by design. You focus on foods that are soft, low in fiber, and easy to digest. In Phase 2, you start adding select new items. It helps to break these options down by food group and highlight why some foods are safe early and others must wait.

Grains and Breads

- **Safe in Phase 1:** Refined white breads, plain crackers (such as saltines or Melba toast), soft white rolls, pancakes made from white flour, plain French toast, and white rice. Cooked cereals like cream of wheat, farina, and grits make the list, as well as dry cereals like corn flakes or puffed rice. Pasta, noodles, and cooked potatoes without skin are also allowed.

- **Wait for Phase 2:** Whole-grain items, brown rice, cereals with bran or seeds, corn bread, graham crackers, and bread or desserts containing dried fruit, seeds, or nuts stay off the menu until good tolerance is proven.

Fruits and Fruit Juices

- **Safe in Phase 1:** Canned or cooked fruits without skins or seeds—think applesauce, canned peaches, or pears. Ripe bananas and soft melons (like cantaloupe and honeydew) also qualify. Strained fruit juice without pulp, such as apple, no-pulp orange, or cranberry, is permitted.
- **Wait for Phase 2:** Raw fruits, berries, pineapple, dried fruits, and juices with pulp need to be postponed. These items tend to leave more residue in your intestines.

Vegetables

- **Safe in Phase 1:** Most well-cooked or canned vegetables as long as they lack seeds and skins. Good choices include cooked carrots, green beans, pumpkins, and winter squash (without seeds). Lettuce can be tried if you know it does not upset you. Strained vegetable juice made from allowed vegetables can fit, too.
- **Wait for Phase 2:** Avoid most raw vegetables, broccoli, cauliflower, cabbage, onions, peas, corn, greens (like kale or Swiss chard), potatoes with skin, and beans during the early stage. These are harder to digest and can quickly bring back symptoms.

Protein Foods (Meats, Eggs, Dairy)

- **Safe in Phase 1:** Tender, well-cooked meats (like ground beef, poultry, ham, pork, veal, or fish). Eggs work well. Cheese and plain yogurt are included for those who tolerate dairy, but avoid versions with nuts, seeds, or fruit added.
- **Wait for Phase 2:** Fibrous meats, gristly cuts, smoked or cured deli options, and meat with tough outer membranes are off-limits. Beans, lentils, dry peas, tofu, and peanut butter must wait, as must any cheese containing fruit or seeds.

Fats, Snack Foods, and Sweets

- **Safe in Phase 1:** Margarine, butter, oils, mayonnaise, sour cream, plain salad dressings, and simple gravies. Plain cakes and cookies, gelatin, custard, ice cream, sherbet, and popsicles can be enjoyed in moderation. Plain hard candy, pretzels (not whole grain), and vanilla wafers are other options.
- **Wait for Phase 2:** Avoid any snack or dessert made with seeds, nuts, dried fruit, whole grains, popcorn, and jam, marmalade, or preserves.

Condiments and Beverages

- **Safe in Phase 1:** Spices, cooked herbs, bouillon, broth (prepared only with allowed foods), decaf coffee or tea, carbonated drinks, strained vegetable juices, and diluted juices made from allowed fruits. Milk is allowed if you tolerate lactose. Otherwise, opt for lactose-free versions or small portions.
- **Wait for Phase 2:** Pickles, olives, relish, sauerkraut, horseradish, and any beverage with seeds, pulp, or strong artificial coloring.

As you move from strict to recovery phases, the main goal is to expand your food choices without causing symptoms to return. Each shift lets you reclaim foods you enjoy, but only as your gut allows.

Food Swaps: Adapting for Vegetarian, Lactose-Free, and Diverse Diets

People rarely eat the exact same foods or have the same dietary needs. Special attention is needed for vegetarians, those with lactose intolerance, and those with varied cultural diets. Here is how you can adapt core recommendations for different lifestyles:

For Vegetarians:

- **In Phase 1,** protein options are slim, since legumes and most nuts are excluded. Lean eggs and dairy (if tolerated) become the default. Soft tofu may be tried once symptoms stabilize and with your provider's guidance, but beans or lentils should be avoided in the strictest period.
- **In Phase 2,** introduce small portions of peeled, well-cooked lentils or split mung beans, pureed if needed, and see how you feel after 24–48 hours. Tofu and smooth nut butters (no crunchy seeds) can also be trialed carefully.
- Soft dairy options, such as cottage cheese, may replace meat as protein sources.

For People with Lactose Intolerance:

- Stick to lactose-free milk, yogurt, and cheese alternatives. Many grocery stores carry lactose-free versions that blend in well where regular dairy is called for.

- Some tolerate hard cheeses (like Swiss or cheddar) in small amounts, as these usually have less lactose.
- If you want to try regular dairy, test a small serving with lactase supplements, paying close attention to your body's reaction.

***For Diverse Cultural Diets*:**

- Many staple foods, such as white rice or refined pasta, are universally acceptable and can act as substitutes for traditional bread or flatbread.
- For East Asian diets, soft white rice and mild broths work well. Avoid kimchi, pickled veggies, or whole seed preparations early on.
- For South Asian menus, plain, peeled potatoes, white rice, thin dal made without whole pulses, and soft paneer may fit later in recovery.
- For Mediterranean preferences, try white bread, clear broths, soft boiled fish, and mild cheeses.
- In Latin American diets, polenta made from degermed corn or finely sifted arepas (without added seeds) can be used.

Smart food swapping is about finding acceptable, gentle alternatives that still deliver joy and nutrition. If you belong to more than one group, say, vegetarian and lactose intolerant, focus on eggs, careful introduction of soft legumes in Phase 2, and lactose-free dairy substitutes.

Flags for Ingredient Addition or Removal

As you start to expand your foods, several clues can guide you on whether to keep going or pause. Work with the following signals:

1. ***Preparation Method***:

Stick to soft, well-cooked, or pureed food preparation, especially when trying any new fruit or vegetable for the first time after a flare. Skins and seeds tend to spark symptoms early on, so always peel and strain as needed. Avoiding fried or heavy, greasy cooking is another smart filter, since high-fat prep can lead to diarrhea or bloating.

1. ***Tolerance***:

Introduce only one new food at a time, starting with a small portion. If you do well over 24–48 hours—no rise in pain, bloating, or loose stools—add it to your "safe" list. If any symptoms return, remove the new food, wait to recover, then try a different option. This slow testing lets you pinpoint personal triggers safely.

2. ***Symptom Feedback***:

Use a log to record what you tried, including amounts and cooking details, and note your body's response afterward. If you have even mild swelling, cramps, or changes in stool, repeat only what's well tolerated or pull back to the prior diet stage.

3. ***Food Quality***:

Even for allowed foods, watch for brands or recipes that quietly add whole grain flours, seeds, or extra fiber as thickeners. Read ingredient lists closely on breads, crackers, and cereals. Variations between brands can make a real difference.

In short, only expand ingredients when meals are gentle in preparation, tried in small amounts, and symptom logs show green lights. The pace may differ between individuals, and readiness can vary week by week.

Connecting Foods to Phase-Specific Advantages and Drawbacks

Each food and cooking approach brings clear pros and cons tied to where you are in your recovery. Here, you will find a charted summary to help link your food selection with expected outcomes.

Phase 1 "Allowed" Foods

- **Refined grains (white bread, rice, pasta):** Soothing, low residue, and rarely problematic. Can sometimes lead to constipation if used without enough fluid.
- **Canned/cooked fruits (without skin/seeds):** Low irritation, good sugar source, but not much fiber or vitamin C.
- **Tender meats, eggs, lactose-free dairy:** Good for protein, but can feel monotonous and exclude plant nutrients. Some cheese may increase bloating for those with mild dairy issues.

Phase 1 "To Avoid"

- **Whole grains, nuts, seeds:** Can trigger pain, cramps, or increased stool, especially in strictures or post-surgical patients.
- **Raw/dried fruits, berries:** Often bring back bloating, gas, or diarrhea.
- **Beans and legumes:** High fiber, often linked to a return of pain or too much gas early on.

Phase 2 "New Additions"

- **Peeled, cooked vegetables:** Most people tolerate peeled sweet potatoes, carrots, and squash well. They restore vitamins and taste.

- **Soft, peeled fruits:** Start with ripe pear halves (canned), peeled apples (in sauce or baked), or banana. Contain more fiber, so introduce slowly.
- **Whole grain items (in small servings):** Encourage gut adaptation and avoid long-term nutritional gaps, but must be introduced carefully. If constipated, these can help, but in high amounts they may return you to pain or swelling.

<u>**Possible Complications:**</u>

- **Dairy items:** In lactose-sensitive people, milk or ice cream can cause cramps or diarrhea. Switch to lactose-free or reduce serving size.
- **Tough meats or fatty foods:** May cause discomfort or slow digestion after surgery or flare. Choose softer cuts and low-fat cooking methods.

<u>**Possible Advantages:**</u>

- **Controlled introduction:** Lessens the risk of symptom relapse.
- **Broadening produce:** Supports better vitamin and mineral intake and reduces constipation risk in the longer term.

Shopping and Stocking Up: Quick Reference and Adaptation Tips

Planning your grocery trip becomes much easier when you know what to look for, both for the strict restriction phase and the gradual re-expansion period. Here's a ready-to-use shopping reference:

<u>***Phase 1 Shopping List Essentials***</u>

- White bread, sandwich rolls, and bagels (without seeds)
- Plain crackers: saltines, Melba toast
- White rice, plain pasta, or noodles
- Cold cereals: corn flakes, puffed rice
- Cooked cereals: cream of wheat, farina
- Canned fruits in juice or light syrup (no skin or seeds)
- Ripe bananas, soft melon
- Well-cooked or canned vegetables: carrots, pumpkin, green beans, squash (no seeds/skins)
- Tender meats: ground beef, skinless poultry, pork, white fish
- Eggs
- Dairy: lactose-free milk, yogurt, hard cheese (if tolerated)
- Margarine, butter, simple salad dressings
- Plain sweets: gelatin, vanilla wafers, plain cookies, ice pops
- Decaf coffee/tea, apple or grape juice (no pulp), strained vegetable broth.

Phase 2 Add-Ons for Gentle Expansion

- Peeled, well-cooked sweet potatoes, peeled white or gold potatoes in small amounts
- Small portions of soft, peeled, cooked fruit (apple, pear)
- Whole grain bread or pasta: introduce 1–2 slices or a small serving each week
- Beans or lentils: start with pureed and peeled, in tiny servings
- Smooth nut or seed butters (if well tolerated)
- Oatmeal or "instant" oats, prepared without extra seeds or fruit

Adaptation Notes:

- Stick to familiar brands if possible, especially when tolerating a food for the first time.
- Stock up on lactose-free or plant-based dairy alternatives before a flare.
- For vegetarians, eggs and permitted dairy are key in early recovery, but check labels to ensure there are no added seeds or excessive fiber.
- For multicultural needs, focus on core starches and permitted proteins that fit your culinary background, modifying recipes so that everything is soft and free of seeds/skins.

It is a wise move to keep a food diary during shopping and meal prep. If a new purchase leads to symptoms, record the brand and type, so you can avoid it next time. When in doubt, ask your provider to review your proposed list or connect you to a registered dietitian for further adaptation.

Meal Flexibility and Ongoing Personalization

Success with a low fiber, low residue eating plan comes from matching structure with flexibility. You build your foundation with core approved foods and only move forward once your system responds well. Adaptation means drawing upon suitable swaps, tailored portion sizes, and careful cooking.

You may find that what works for one person in Phase 1 causes another trouble; for example, soft white wheat bread may digest easily for you but not for someone with gluten intolerance. Your tolerance for certain foods will likely improve so keep an up-to-date list of personal safe options and stay open to adding new items in small, controlled tests.

The food lists and ingredient expansions covered here form the backbone of a successful flare recovery or post-surgical transition. Return to these as your needs change, and involve your care team when a food or preparation method leaves you uncertain. Equipped with these frameworks and clear phase-specific grids, you can shop, prepare, and adapt meals confidently for both effective symptom relief and satisfying variety.

Nutritional Management and Preventing Deficiencies

Health professionals know that following a low fiber, low residue diet can provide symptom relief, but it often comes at the cost of nutrition and that cost rises the longer strict food limits are in place. With so many foods off the table, patients may feel they walk a nutritional tightrope, especially for vitamins, minerals, and protein.

The question is not just what you must give up, but how you can guard against shortfalls and keep your body strong during each phase. To meet this challenge, you need targeted strategies that go beyond basic lists: you require a practical plan for identifying your risks, maintaining a balanced intake, and knowing how and when to seek expert support.

A new symptom may arise, or your energy could dip just when meal planning feels hardest. The solution lies in understanding which nutrients are at risk (and when), practical ways to protect your daily intake, and how to spot less obvious sources of fiber or residue in everyday foods. Instead of letting deficiencies creep up, you can use structured guidance and careful observation to stay ahead of these problems.

Assessing Nutrient Risks in Both Diet Phases

Each phase of this diet brings its own nutritional threats. During the strictest periods, choices are limited, and many high-value foods disappear. When you expand the menu, some risks lessen—but others may linger if variety does not increase. This is why seeing nutrient risk as a spectrum helps you make smart, timely adjustments.

For a quick overview, the following table summarizes common nutrients at risk during both diet phases, with each risk grouped by phase and color-coded for practical action:

Phase 1 (Strict):

- **High Risk**: Fiber, vitamin C, folate, potassium, magnesium, vitamin K
- **Moderate Risk**: Calcium (if low dairy or lactose intolerant), vitamin D, protein (for vegetarians or those with low appetite)
- **Low Risk**: Iron and B vitamins (if some meat, eggs included), sodium (usually not an issue due to processed foods).

Phase 2 (Early Recovery):

- **Moderate Risk**: Fiber (unless whole grains/vegetables return), vitamin C, folate
- **Low Risk**: Protein, calcium, iron (most rebalanced with careful expansion), vitamin D (with some sun or supplements); magnesium and potassium (rise only if produce and legumes stay limited).

Red means nutrients most at risk that need quick attention.

Yellow suggests moderate watchfulness, especially if your intake pattern stays narrow.

Green indicates the lowest concern when core food groups are included.

If you must follow the diet longer than two weeks, speak with your provider about a daily multivitamin with minerals and whether you require any other supplements.

Every person enters the diet with a different health background. Previous surgeries, medication use, and baseline nutrition play a role in these risks. Keeping your food and symptom log is key to noticing gaps early and supporting recovery.

Building Protein, Vitamin, and Mineral Intake Under Restrictions

The shift to a low fiber, low residue diet does not have to mean giving up on quality nutrition. Rather, success depends on creative reinforcement strategies across both phases. Instead of waiting for signs of low energy or slow healing, you can take steps each day to maintain your intake within the limits of the diet.

These reinforcement tactics can help:

- **Choose protein-rich soft foods:** Eggs, tender meats, plain fish, and permitted dairy (like lactose-free milk, yogurt, and hard cheeses) offer a strong base during Phase 1. Prioritize these at each meal. If you do not eat meat, lean on eggs and permitted cheeses, and consider soft tofu or well-poured legumes only once your symptoms improve and with professional advice.

- **Maximize your use of canned or well-cooked fruits and vegetables:** Soft forms preserve some vitamins and minerals, including potassium and vitamin C, though levels are lower than in raw produce. Include these foods daily when allowed in your phase, and always peel or strain anything with skin, pulp, or seeds.
- **If you tolerate dairy, use it for calcium and vitamin D:** Aim for two servings per day if possible, even if it means using lactose-free options. These also help add protein and some B vitamins.
- **Use a food diary:** Write down what you eat over at least a week. Note how each food makes you feel and how often you can include protein, fruits, and vegetables. This helps spot patterns and keeps you accountable for daily variety.
- **Pay attention to fluid intake:** Many foods on this diet contain less water and fiber, which can slow digestion. Drinking enough low-residue fluids (clear broths, water, some juices) helps keep things moving and supports kidney and vitamin C balance.
- **Rotate approved snacks to avoid boredom and boost energy:** Plain cookies or gelatin desserts may sound bland, but when paired with fruit puree or yogurt, they deliver more nutrition. Hard candy offers simple calories, which can be useful for those struggling with appetite.
- **Set reminders to eat every 3–4 hours:** Skipping meals is common if appetite lags, but regular spacing helps support steady nutrient intake. If mornings are hard, start with a small amount,

half a banana or a spoonful of custard then build up as hunger returns.

Some days you may hit every food group; on other days, you might repeat the same protein. The diary helps you see which foods help maintain your intake and which ones cause symptoms, so you can adapt quickly.

Supplementation Guide for Short- and Long-Term Use

Supplements can serve as a bridge when gaps persist, but you need to use them wisely and only when markers call for it. Not every bottle suits your exact needs under gastrointestinal stress, and some forms—like those containing extra fiber or residue—may harm more than help. Safe supplement use comes down to a few key questions.

Has your provider advised that you stay on the diet longer than two weeks? If so, a standard multivitamin with minerals is recommended to fill most shortfalls. Make sure it does not contain added fiber or herbs, as these can disrupt the balance you are trying to achieve.

Are you experiencing symptoms of a specific deficiency—fatigue, muscle cramps, prolonged wound healing, or new hair loss? If these appear, request a lab assessment to pinpoint which nutrients are low and ask for professional advice before starting extra single-nutrient (e.g., iron, calcium, vitamin D) supplements.

Read supplement ingredient lists closely. Products marketed for 'digestive health' sometimes add gums, inulin, psyllium, or fruit powders for texture. These are not suitable for low fiber, low residue diets.

Use supplements within the following boundaries:

- **Daily multivitamin with minerals:** Use only if diet lasts more than two weeks or if dietary variety is minimal.
- **Calcium, vitamin D, and iron:** Only add after provider review of your intake and, if needed, blood levels. Too much can cause constipation or mask underlying gastrointestinal issues.
- **Protein powders:** Not generally needed unless intake is very low and appetite is suppressed, and only after checking the product for hidden fiber or added ingredients.
- **Electrolyte solutions or beverages:** Acceptable if symptoms suggest significant loss (vomiting, diarrhea), but avoid those containing pulp, fiber, or insoluble additives.

Supplements are not substitutes for meals; they serve as a stopgap while you work to improve food variety as symptoms ease.

Reading Labels to Spot Hidden Fiber or Residue

Packaged foods do not always reveal their secrets at a glance. Many processed items, especially those that market themselves as "healthy," include hidden sources of fiber, whole grains, seeds, or dried fruit—even in foods that would appear benign, like bread, cereal, or crackers. Mastering label review will keep these from sneaking into your diet and causing setbacks.

Here's how to scan and decode a food label and ingredient list for hidden sources of fiber and residue:

- **Begin with the ingredient list, not just the Nutrition Facts panel.** Look for the first few ingredients and avoid those that mention whole wheat, bran, seeds, nuts, or dried fruits. Labels often hide extra fiber as "inulin," "psyllium," "fibra," or "chicory root."
- **For breads and crackers, confirm that only refined white flour is used;** avoid any version with visible grains, oats, or mention of "whole grain." Words like multigrain, 7-grain, or sprouted indicate unfit options.
- **In cereals, spot additions like "bran," "wheat germ," "raisins," or "nuts."** Even cereals that are mostly puffed rice or corn sometimes contain clusters or flakes made from whole grains or dried fruit pieces.
- **Yogurt or dairy items should be plain and free of seeds, coconut, or fruit-on-the-bottom.** Choose only those with minimal ingredients: milk, cream, live cultures. Skip those with sprinkles, granola add-ins, or mix-ins containing nuts or fruit bits.
- **Canned fruits and prepared desserts deserve scrutiny for fruit skin, seeds, or added bulkers made from natural fibers.** Labels may include additives for thickening, like "modified food starch" (usually safe) but should not list actual fiber blends or pureed skins.
- **Condiments should be free from visible seeds** (like mustard, relish, or pickled products) and avoid any product listing "ground flaxseed," "chia," or "tomato skin puree".

When label language is unclear, select the simplest version available—plain white versions of bread, rice, and noodles, or clear juices with "strained" or "without pulp" prominently shown on the packaging.

Getting Support: When to See a Registered Dietitian and Personalizing Your Plan

Certain symptoms signal the need for a professional review, and keeping notes (or using a worksheet) helps you decide when a consult is wise. While most adults can self-manage daily choices for a few weeks, some situations require more careful review.

Triggers for a registered dietitian consult include:

- Extended use of the dietary restrictions (beyond two weeks)
- Ongoing or worsening symptoms (bloating, pain, diarrhea, unexpected weight loss)
- Difficulties in maintaining or regaining weight
- Repeat GI flares without clear cause, especially after food expansion
- Visible nutrient deficiency symptoms: fatigue, loss of strength, mouth ulcers, hair thinning, dry skin, poor wound healing
- Trouble finding approved foods that match medical, allergy, cultural, or lifestyle needs
- Complex medical conditions or medication use that affects nutrient needs or absorption

To help with ongoing personalization, build a worksheet (either with a dietitian or on your own) with these guiding columns:

1. Core foods I can tolerate (by group: grains, fruits, vegetables, proteins, fats, dairy)
2. Current phase and list of foods I hope to add (with room for symptom notes)
3. Nutrient targets I worry about (based on the colored table above)
4. Current supplements taken (dose, frequency, date started)
5. Symptoms noticed since last food expansion or supplement change
6. Questions for next appointment or email to dietitian/provider

Filling out this tool every week or after any dietary change keeps your adjustment process responsive and protects against silent deficiencies. Bringing the worksheet and your detailed food log to each provider visit lets your team offer much more specific feedback and helps them fine-tune your plan.

Nutritional management in a low fiber, low residue protocol is about more than following rules; it requires active prevention of shortfalls at every step. When you know which nutrients require special vigilance, reinforce your intake with approved foods, review supplements with care, and read every label for hidden pitfalls, you dramatically reduce the chance for slow declines or costly mistakes.

Most adults benefit from a careful, organized approach—supported by tracking logs, structured intake rotation, and clear points when professional guidance is best sought. Through this kind of vigilance, your diet remains a tool for healing, not a risk to recovery.

If challenges come up, ask for help from your provider. Partnering with a dietitian ensures your choices are right for your needs and supports you through the complexities of both symptom control and nutritional adequacy. With the frameworks, strategies, and consult triggers above, you can stay on the best path toward symptom relief, safe food expansion, and ongoing health.

Cooking Methods, Textural Adaptations, and Safe Meal Prep

Choosing effective ways to prepare meals on a low fiber, low residue diet can help prevent discomfort or a return of symptoms. Many adults feel lost when moving away from familiar foods, but the right cooking strategies help preserve both nutrition and eating pleasure even with common restrictions.

This chapter approaches meal preparation not as a simple list of instructions, but as a process of matching methods, tools, and textures to individual needs at every phase. It explains each step, shares which kitchen essentials truly help, and demonstrates how to keep food safe and appealing over repeat meals.

Matching Cooking Methods to Food Groups and Phases

Choosing how to cook and prepare food shapes both digestion and enjoyment. In the strictest phase, only the gentlest methods work. As your tolerance improves or your provider allows expansion, new methods become possible. The following practical guide connects cooking methods directly to the main food groups found on this diet:

1. **Soft grains:** Boiling is ideal for white rice, refined noodles, and pasta. Cooking them until very tender, even beyond "al

dente," makes them easier to digest. Steaming can work for those who want to cook multiple items together using minimal fat and no fiber-boosting ingredients. For breakfast grains such as farina or cream of wheat, simmering in extra water until soft creates a smooth texture.

2. **Vegetables:** Steaming and boiling without skins are the most reliable. These methods break down vegetable fibers so they are gentler on the gut. Well-cooked carrots, green beans, beets, spinach, zucchini, pumpkin, and winter squash without seeds are all suitable if soft and peeled. Some people prefer baking, but the food must reach a mashable consistency. Pureeing with a little fluid can further reduce any remaining solids.
3. **Fruits:** Poaching, baking, or simmering turn canned or fresh seedless, skinless fruits into gentle options. Applesauce and canned pears, for example, are best served very soft. For denser fruits, such as pumpkin, baking until soft then removing any skin and pureeing is safe.
4. **Proteins:** Baking, broiling, or poaching works well for chicken, turkey, and fish. Moist heat helps prevent toughness. For meats, shaving or slicing very thin after cooking aids swallowing and digestibility. Scrambled eggs need only a quick, gentle cook to become soft and easy to digest.
5. **Potatoes:** Only peeled, boiled or baked without skin are recommended. Mash well for the softest texture. Avoid frying, as it adds fat and may cause discomfort.
6. **Approved dairy:** Milk, custard, and soft cheeses often require only gentle heating or blending into dishes. Yogurt

must be plain and free of seeds or fruit bits. Use low heat to create puddings or custards.

7. **Sweets:** Plain cakes, cookies, gelatin, and puddings are best made with refined flours. Baking works as long as there are no seeds, nuts, or whole-grain add-ins. Many plain desserts tolerate moderate baking without changing their low-residue status.

Each food group connects to a set of methods that maximize tolerability. Steaming, boiling, poaching, and pureeing are the safest choices in Phase 1. As tolerance improves, typically in Phase 2, baking and broiling can be added if foods remain tender and digestion stays comfortable.

Kitchen Tools and Safe Preparation for Digestible Meals

A well-planned kitchen setup makes meal prep on a restricted diet less tiring, more efficient, and safer. Not every gadget is needed, but several key items can make a big difference.

1. **Peeler:** A strong peeler quickly removes skins from vegetables and fruits, such as carrots, potatoes, apples, and pears. Removing rough skins is non-negotiable for lowering fiber and residue.
2. **Fine mesh strainer or sieve:** Use for draining canned fruits and vegetables, rinsing small pasta shapes, or straining seeds and pulp from juices or soups.

3. **Sharp knife and cutting board:** A sharp, comfortable knife billed as "vegetable" or "utility" ensures safe handling when slicing soft, peeled produce or tender meats.
4. **Potato masher or sturdy fork:** For mashing cooked vegetables and potatoes into smooth consistency. This is especially valuable for people in the strictest phase or with chewing difficulties.
5. **Small food processor or hand blender:** Not required, but very helpful for pureeing foods to a near-liquid texture. A mini chopper can also make finely chopped meats, vegetables, or soft fruits safer to swallow.
6. **Saucepan and steamer basket:** These allow for moist heat cooking of vegetables, fruits, and grains. Steamer baskets keep nutrients in the food and permit batch cooking of several items at once.
7. **Measuring spoons and cups:** Useful for precise portioning, especially to keep meals small enough for easy digestion and to help track nutritional intake as advised in earlier chapters.

Safe meal preparation also means being mindful of cross-contamination and cleanliness. Always use separate boards and utensils for raw meats and ready-to-eat foods. Wash produce with running water before peeling, and clean all tools thoroughly after each use. Soft foods may spoil quickly, so refrigerate leftovers within two hours. If reheating later, heat foods until they are steaming and serve immediately. Do not refreeze thawed cooked meals.

Texture and Digestibility: Stepwise Adaptation in Practice

Altering food texture can make a significant difference in tolerability for people following strict diets. A gradual, three-stage approach works well for most solid foods on this plan.

Begin by removing the skins from raw produce before cooking, as the outer layers of apples, potatoes, and carrots contain most of the fiber that can trigger digestive issues. For some fruits and vegetables, briefly parboiling helps loosen the skin for easier peeling.

Cook the peeled produce until it reaches a very soft consistency—boil or steam grains and vegetables, or bake or poach soft fruits. The goal is a texture soft enough to mash easily with a fork. Incorporating water or broth helps maintain a moist, shapeable consistency. If introducing new foods or during periods of digestive sensitivity, add additional moisture and sample a small amount to check for tolerability.

After cooking, mash or puree as needed. Use a potato masher for soft, cooked vegetables, and for a smoother result, try a food processor or hand blender, blending until completely smooth. When preparing meats, slice thinly, shred, or mince after cooking to make proteins easier to digest. Divide foods into small portions using cups or containers for gentle, convenient meals that cool quickly for storage.

A food diary can help identify which textures are best tolerated and when it might be time to try thicker or more solid foods.

Introducing one new texture at a time and monitoring for symptoms throughout the day supports a more successful transition.

Flavor Boosts Without Extra Residue or Discomfort

Enjoyment matters for long-term adherence to restricted diets. While whole herbs, spicy sauces, or chunky salsas must be avoided, there are ways to bring excitement and freshness to bland meals without risking symptoms.

1. **Use permitted fats:** Small amounts of butter, margarine, olive oil, or even mayonnaise add flavor and moisture to grains, protein, and soft vegetables. A dab of sour cream or cream cheese can soften the feel of a baked potato or scrambled eggs.
2. **Smooth condiments:** Smooth salad dressing, plain mayonnaise, honey, clear jellies (without seeds), maple syrup, or simple gravies give roundness to dishes without texture hazards. Avoid chunky, seeded, or fibrous spreads.
3. **Mild spices and cooked herbs:** Bouillon, broth, or soups made with permitted ingredients provide both flavor and hydration. Use strained or well-cooked herbs (such as parsley or chives) in small amounts. Avoid any visible stems, seeds, or large herb pieces.
4. **Broths and flavored liquids:** These can be sipped plain or used when cooking grains, vegetables, or proteins to infuse background notes of flavor.

5. **Acidic accents:** A squeeze of lemon juice or a dash of vinegar (strained) can brighten dishes. Make sure acidic condiments are free from pulp.
6. **Desserts and soft sweets:** Vanilla and almond extracts, when added to custards, gelatins, plain puddings, or ice cream, boost interest and sweetness without harsh textures or extra residue.

Vary flavors between meals, even when using the same core ingredient, to keep meals appealing. For example, plain white rice at lunch can be savory with a little butter and broth, then served as a sweet pudding at dinner with milk and a touch of honey.

Safe Meal Prep, Batch Cooking, and Storage for Restricted Diets

For many adults, energy and motivation run low during dietary restriction or symptom flares. Batch cooking turns one afternoon of work into several days of meals and reduces the daily burden of food decisions. The key is to maintain safety at each step and store foods in a way that doesn't increase risk.

Plan meals in advance, focusing on 2–3 types of protein, 2–3 safe grains, 3–4 soft vegetables, and 2–3 permitted fruits. Write a simple list, then convert it into a plan for reheating and serving over a few days.

1. **Cook all foods until very tender.** Peel and remove any skins and visible seeds from produce before cooking. Use separate

utensils for raw and cooked items. This prevents accidental transfer of bacteria.

2. **Divide finished dishes into single-serving containers for easy portion control and quick reheating.** Label each container with the contents and the date it was prepared.
3. **Cool food and refrigerate within two hours.** Do not leave foods at room temperature, as bacterial growth happens more quickly in soft, protein-rich and moist foods. Use shallow containers so food chills fast.
4. **Store cooked meals on a front shelf in the refrigerator.** Safe storage times for most cooked meats, soft grains, and pureed vegetables is up to three days. Canned fruits and other low risk items, once opened, should be used within three days as well.
5. **Reheat thoroughly.** Foods must be heated until steaming throughout before eating, even if only a small portion is needed. Avoid reheating more than once if possible; repeated heating and cooling can raise the risk of spoilage.
6. **If freezing, divide food into small portions so you can thaw only what you need.** Thaw in the refrigerator—not on the counter—to keep risk of bacterial growth minimal. Reheat from frozen until piping hot.
7. **For beverages, store only what you will use in 2–3 days, especially if fruit juices or non-dairy milks are included; these can sour quickly.** Juices should always be pulp-free and, if possible, strained again before serving.

Batch cooking works best when menus feature a repeating set of soft, safe foods. For example, you can prepare a tray of baked chicken breast, a pot of white rice, and three vegetable sides such as peeled carrots, green beans, and canned spinach. Mix and match servings throughout the week, adding different permitted sauces or flavorings to keep things interesting. A few easy snacks (plain crackers, vanilla pudding) can be portioned ahead so there is always something gentle on hand.

A meal plan and tracked rotation of flavors and foods support both nutrition and mental satisfaction, especially when eating the same foods several days in a row.

Sample Troubleshooting Scenarios for Meal Prep and Adaptation

Sometimes, things do not go as planned. Reviewing common issues can help adults maintain both safety and pleasure in food during restricted periods.

If cooked grains or vegetables feel gritty or have bits, process further with more fluid to achieve a truly smooth texture. Strain if needed to ensure no skin or seed fragments remain.

Should a meal trigger discomfort, review your steps: Was every skin or seed removed? Was the food cooked until truly soft? Did you try a new condiment or flavor that could cause irritation? Use your food diary to pinpoint changes that may bother your gut. If unsure, revert to a simpler previous version and advance when symptoms permit.

If running out of ideas, rotate the core proteins and grains by preparation method: grill chicken one day and poach it the next, or alternate between plain rice and pasta. Small textural and flavor shifts within the safe limits reduce boredom while still guarding against symptoms.

If appetite wanes, try assembling smaller, snack-style meals several times a day. Soft puddings, mild broths, and mashed fruits foster steady intake for days when full meals feel impossible.

Contact a healthcare provider or dietitian if you are unable to keep meals varied, safe, and satisfying.

Effective cooking and meal preparation on a low fiber, low residue diet rely on a few central strategies: using the right gentle methods (steaming, boiling, baking), matching kitchen tools and storage flow to your current abilities, phasing texture changes for comfort and absorption, boosting flavor without residue, and planning ahead for safe and quick meals. Each step can help you keep food safe, meals enjoyable, and nutrient intake steady—no matter how strict your current eating phase or how long your recovery takes.

These skills build resilience and bring back some agency to everyday eating, even when ingredients are few. Learning these techniques can make living with food limitations more manageable and less stressful. With structure, creativity, and a willingness to adapt, you are well equipped to handle the ongoing challenges of a restricted diet and support your digestive healing from the kitchen out.

Meal Plans and Adaptable Templates for Diverse Needs

Dietary adaptation during digestive recovery requires more than knowing which foods are allowed. It means finding a routine that fits your individual needs and context. Set meal patterns and formulaic menus are only as helpful as their flexibility. People with different schedules, tastes, economic backgrounds, and levels of kitchen skill all need a model they can shape to their specific situation.

This chapter focuses on providing practical, actionable meal templates that can be mixed, adapted, and reworked to suit real-world demands, while maintaining the nutritional safeguards needed for digestive healing.

The key to successful nourishment on a low fiber, low residue diet lies in reducing guesswork and decision fatigue while leaving room for individual difference. Many adults experience frustration moving between strict and less strict phases—what seems soothing one week becomes unappealing or even triggering the next. Strong meal planning templates, clear portion guidance, and visual tools that explain both macros and micronutrients help restore a sense of control over food choices, even when many options feel off-limits.

A 7-Day Rotating Meal Template for Each Diet Phase

A rotating meal framework takes the mental load off decision-making and supports steady nutrition through the variety a week can offer. This plan can be used as a foundation for both strict (Phase 1) and more liberal (Phase 2) periods of the low residue diet. Each day's pattern maintains consistent timing and portion guidance to ease digestion and avoid large, difficult-to-handle meals.

For adults in the strict phase, start with these fundamentals:

Breakfast:

- 1 cup of a soft, cooked cereal such as farina or cream of wheat. Serve with 1/2 cup of lactose-free or regular milk (if tolerated).
- 1 scrambled egg for protein.
- 1 slice of refined white toast with margarine and smooth jelly (no seeds).
- 1 cup of a pulp-free juice, such as apple or cranberry.

Lunch:

- Baked or poached chicken, about 2–3 ounces, with 1/2 cup of white rice.
- 1/2 cup of canned or well-cooked carrots or green beans, drained.
- White dinner roll with butter or margarine.
- 1/2 cup smooth pudding or plain yogurt if dairy is tolerated.

Snack (optional if energy needs are higher):

- 1 soft cake or vanilla wafer.

- 1/2 cup pulp-free juice.

Dinner:

- 2–3 ounces of baked or tender roast beef or fish.
- 1/2 cup white rice or mashed potatoes with no skin.
- 1/2 cup well-cooked spinach or canned green beans.
- 1 white dinner roll with soft margarine.

Throughout the day:

- Safe beverages include decaffeinated coffee or tea with sugar and a splash of milk, as tolerated. Hydration can be supplemented by strained clear broths.

Rotate in alternate grains like plain white pasta, expand the protein to soft fish, and use permitted desserts such as gelatin, puddings, or vanilla ice cream for variety during the week.

In Phase 2, as more tolerance develops, you can include lean ham, tender turkey, or well-cooked, peeled vegetables such as peeled zucchini or squash. If well-tolerated, lettuces can be tried in small amounts in a salad with smooth dressing. Fruits can be expanded to canned fruits in juice or applesauce, provided skins and seeds are fully removed.

Portion guidance remains steady: main protein servings of 2–3 ounces per meal, each starch at 1/2 to 1 cup, and vegetables or fruits at 1/2 cup. Always test new additions in single servings for at least a day before repeating.

Texture cues matter: every item should be easily mashable with a fork. Foods must remain moist, soft, and free of tough or stringy bits. Return to the stricter meal plan if any symptoms appear.

Plug-and-Play Meal Builder Blocks

Some days may not fit a fixed plan. Job changes, family preferences, or sudden changes in appetite can derail even the best intentions. Rather than forcing every meal into an exact format, use building blocks that allow you to swap, combine, or simplify as needed.

Base starches (choose one per meal):

- White rice, mashed white potatoes (no skin), soft pasta, or cream of wheat.
- For economic or cultural adaptations, plain white corn grits or soft polenta (if well-cooked and strained) can stand in.

Proteins (choose one per meal):

- Scrambled or softly boiled eggs.
- Well-cooked, peeled, boneless chicken, turkey, lean ground beef, or mild fish like tilapia or cod.
- Vegetarian swap: Silken tofu gently steamed or mashed, or lactose-free plain yogurt if animal protein must be avoided (avoid nuts, seeds, and unstrained legumes).

Vegetable sides (choose up to two in small servings):

- Canned green beans, carrots, beets, or peeled zucchini—always boiled or steamed until very soft.
- For acid balance or cultural context, try peeled pumpkin or strained tomato sauce on white pasta (if no seed or skin fragments remain).

Fruits (choose for snacks or dessert):

- Canned pears, peaches, applesauce (no peel or skin).

- Banana, if tolerated, only in small, fully ripened pieces and mashed for easier digestion.

Permitted fats and extras:

- Margarine, butter, small drizzles of olive oil, mayonnaise if tolerated.
- Sour cream, plain gravies, or smooth condiments in moderation.

Dairy modifications:

- Use lactose-free milk or fortified non-dairy beverages for those with lactose intolerance.
- For creamy textures, plain custard or smooth non-dairy pudding works as substitutes.

Snack builder:

- Plain pretzels (not whole grain), soft white bread, vanilla wafers.
- Smooth puddings and gelatin (avoiding anything with seeds or whole grains).

Beverages:

- Herbal teas, decaffeinated coffee, pulp-free fruit juice, or clear strained vegetable broth.

These blocks allow family members to customize their meals. For example, serve baked chicken, white rice, and green beans as the base: one person can top the chicken with a bit of lemon juice, while another might prefer it plain. For vegetarians, swap the meat for silken tofu with the same starch and vegetable. Lactose-intolerant individuals use non-dairy alternatives across the plan.

Serving and Substitution Table for Cultural, Economic, and Accessibility Differences

Maintaining familiar eating patterns can ease the psychological strain of strict diets. A serving and substitution table lets you swap core foods while guarding against residue overload or relapse.

Grains:

- **Standard:** White rice, refined pasta, white bread.
- **Economic swap:** Store-brand plain bagels or enriched buns.
- **Cultural swap:** White millet porridge (African), congee (Asian), or grits (Southern US), as long as all are strained and well-cooked.

Proteins:

- **Standard:** Poached chicken, turkey, or lean beef.
- **Economic swap:** Canned chicken (packed in water), deli-sliced turkey (low sodium), or softly poached eggs.
- **Vegetarian swap:** Silken tofu, soft scrambled eggs, smooth plain yogurt (lactose-free if needed).

Vegetables:

- **Standard:** Canned carrots, green beans, or spinach.
- **Economic swap:** Discount or generic canned varieties.
- **Cultural swap:** Soft-cooked chayote (Latin American), well-cooked peeled eggplant (Mediterranean/South Asian), or peeled pumpkin.

Fruits:

- **Standard:** Applesauce, canned pears.

- **Economic swap:** Fruit cocktail in juice, generic-brand applesauce (ensure no added fiber).
- **Cultural swap:** Mashed ripe papaya (tropical), peeled lychee (Asian), or pureed guava, where cost and access allow.

<u>**Fats and condiments:**</u>

- **Standard:** Margarine, plain mayonnaise.
- **Economic swap:** Store-brand margarine or vegetable oil.
- **Cultural swap:** Small amount of ghee (clarified butter) in Indian meals.

<u>**Dairy:**</u>

- **Standard:** Milk or yogurt.
- **Economic swap:** Powdered milk (if reconstituted) or store-brand yogurt.
- **Substitution:** Fortified oat, soy, or rice beverages for those avoiding lactose or animal products.

<u>**Snacks and desserts:**</u>

- **Standard:** Plain cake, cookies, gelatin.
- **Economic swap:** Store-brand vanilla wafers or local, plain sweet breads (if seed and whole grain free).
- **Cultural swap:** Steamed rice cakes (without added coconut or seeds).

Adapting a recipe often comes down to cost and availability. When swapping, the goal is to keep texture, moisture, and digestibility in line with the core diet. Watch for hidden seeds, skins, or whole grains in lower-cost or non-standard foods—these can quietly add residue and trigger symptoms.

Illustrating Nutritional Goals on a Plate: Visual Guidance

Understanding what your plate should look like each meal can simplify planning and boost confidence. For each meal, aim to fill your plate, tray, or bowl using a simple visual ratio that covers energy, protein, and micronutrient needs while avoiding roughage:

- **Half the plate:** Soft, low-residue starch. White rice, pasta, soft white bread, or mashed potatoes supply easy-to-digest carbohydrates and calories needed for rebuilding.
- **One quarter:** Tender protein. This could be a thin slice of baked chicken, a scoop of eggs, or a serving of silken tofu. Each piece should be moist and soft; fat content can be modest if tolerated to aid in texture.
- **One quarter:** Soft vegetable or fruit. Think of a mound of canned carrots, soft green beans, or applesauce. Always avoid raw, seeded, or skin-on vegetables at this stage; everything should be smooth and moist.
- **Side dish or cup:** Dairy or dairy alternative. Provides calcium, vitamin D, and sometimes protein, depending on the item. If drinking milk upsets your stomach, use lactose-free milk or fortified alternatives.
- **Fat accent:** A small dab of margarine, butter, or a teaspoon of oil on grain or vegetable items can improve calorie intake and enjoyment.

This visual spread keeps the main nutrition categories in proportion, even as specific foods may turn over based on tolerance or availability. When symptoms ease, you can try increasing the vegetable or protein portion slightly, but do not add raw or whole-grain items until you are certain they are tolerated.

To cover micronutrients, use a daily multivitamin if your care team recommends it, as the restriction of raw fruits, whole grains, and some vegetables may lead to shortfalls over time.

Meal Tracking Sheet for Symptom Response and Menu Adaptation

Living with fluctuating digestive symptoms means adaptation must be quick and based on real feedback, not guesswork. Keeping a meal tracking sheet is practical for isolating what works and spotting which foods may be problematic. Unlike general food diaries, your tracking sheet should include food choices, texture details, serving size, and any symptoms experienced up to several hours later. With consistency, this allows you and your care team to fine-tune food options safely.

A basic sheet could feature the following columns:

- Date and meal time
- Foods and beverages consumed (be specific: "scrambled egg with margarine" instead of "egg")
- Texture (soft, pureed, mashed, fork-mashable, smooth drink)
- Portion estimate (cups, ounces, or pieces)
- Symptoms noticed (bloating, pain, change in stool, heartburn, etc.)

- Notes on substitutions or flavor changes (tried new brand, swapped tofu for chicken, etc.)

Here's how a few days might look:

<u>Day 1:</u>

Lunch: Baked chicken (3 oz, fork-tender), mashed potatoes with 1 tsp butter (1/2 cup), canned carrots (1/2 cup). **Texture:** all soft, no pieces. Symptom: mild fullness, no discomfort.

<u>Day 2:</u>

Snack: Gelatin dessert (1/2 cup), applesauce (1/2 cup), herbal tea. Texture: smooth. Symptom: no change.

<u>Day 3:</u>

Dinner: White rice (1 cup), soft-cooked fish (2 oz), vanilla pudding (1/2 cup). Rice is less soft than usual. **Symptom:** mild bloating.

This pattern allows you to spot which textures or foods increase symptoms and what combinations seem easiest. Over time, it becomes clear which items to favor, which to trial others, and when to pause new introductions.

Families and caregivers can review this chart to help prepare safe meals, while healthcare providers can use it to recommend tailored changes or spot nutritional gaps. Adapting menus becomes a science, not just guesswork.

A meal plan on a low fiber, low residue diet cannot stay static. Life, taste, symptom variability, and accessibility all require tools beyond a rigid plan. With week-long meal templates to relieve planning stress, building blocks for adaptation, direct swaps for real-world differences, visual meal guidance, and a robust tracking record, you are positioned to manage your nutrition needs effectively and consistently.

Allow yourself permission to flex between structure and creativity within safe diet boundaries, drawing on the food, cultural, and economic realities facing your household. Stay attentive to the feedback your body provides through symptoms and tracking, and adjust at a pace that honors both healing and variety. In time, managing meal rotation, adapting textures, and substituting across diverse needs will become second nature, supporting not just physical recovery, but confidence and comfort at the table.

Easy Recipes and Practical Application Guide

Choosing what to eat when your digestive system is fragile requires more than just a list of safe foods. It involves practical, day-to-day decisions about which dishes feel inviting, can be adapted in a hurry, and still support your recovery. In this chapter, practical use is at the heart of the approach.

Each featured recipe is tagged for its place in the recovery phases, mapped to potential substitutions, and accompanied by clear preparation and troubleshooting instructions. Rather than building static routines, this chapter provides the tools to cook with confidence and react quickly to symptoms or changes in what you can tolerate.

Let's step into a real kitchen, following the path from planning and shopping through adjustment and troubleshooting. All recipes are designed for gentle digestion and easy adaptation, letting you meet both comfort and nutritional needs, even when symptoms are unpredictable. The recipes, swaps, cooking tips, portioning guidance, and tolerance troubleshooting you find here are crafted from evidence-based sources and real-world experience.

Phase-Tagged Recipes: Breakfasts, Mains, Sides, and Snacks

Selecting the right dish starts with understanding where you are in your healing process. Each recipe below notes if it is best suited for Phase 1 (strict symptom control) or Phase 2 (gentle reintroduction).

Breakfast: Creamy Farina with Banana (Phase 1 and Phase 2)

Ingredients:

- 1/4 cup farina (cream of wheat) cereal
- 1 cup lactose-free milk (or water if avoiding dairy)
- Pinch of salt
- 1 teaspoon sugar or honey (skip honey for infants)
- 1/2 ripe banana, mashed (optional in Phase 1, encouraged in Phase 2)

Instructions:

1. In a small saucepan, bring milk (or water) and salt to a gentle simmer over medium heat.
2. Slowly whisk in the farina, stirring to prevent lumps.
3. Continue to stir until the mixture thickens and the grains are soft—about 3–5 minutes.
4. Remove from heat, stir in sugar or honey.
5. For extra calories, add a small dab of butter or margarine.
6. Once cool enough, stir in the mashed banana if tolerated and tolerated in your current phase.
7. Serve warm, making sure the texture is smooth and easy to swallow.

Adaptation notes: In Phase 1, skip bananas unless you have shown tolerance. For lactose intolerance, always use lactose-free milk or water. To increase calories, add up to 2 teaspoons of a permitted fat.

Main: Baked Tender Chicken and Rice (Phase 1 and Phase 2)

Ingredients:

- 1 chicken breast, skinless and boneless
- 1 cup cooked white rice
- 1 tablespoon olive oil or margarine
- Salt (just a pinch)
- 1/2 cup canned or well-cooked carrots, drained

Instructions:

1. Preheat the oven to 350°F (175°C).
2. Place the chicken breast in a baking dish and brush with olive oil (or drizzle margarine).
3. Sprinkle lightly with salt.
4. Cover the dish tightly with foil to keep the chicken moist and bake for 30–35 minutes until chicken is fork-tender and juices run clear.
5. Meanwhile, cook white rice as directed on package instructions, taking care to use plenty of water for maximum softness.
6. Prepare carrots by draining and warming them, or boiling fresh carrots until you can easily mash them with a fork.
7. Serve sliced chicken atop the rice, with soft carrots on the side.

Adaptation notes: In Phase 1, cut the chicken into small, easy-to-chew pieces. For economic swaps, replace fresh chicken with canned, rinsed chicken. To adapt protein, use silken tofu chunks, steamed and drizzled with oil for vegetarians.

Side: White Bread Toast with Grape Jelly (Phase 1, Phase 2 if still tolerated)

Ingredients:

- 1 slice refined white bread
- 1 teaspoon margarine
- 1 teaspoon smooth grape jelly (no seeds)

Instructions:

1. Toast the bread lightly until golden but still soft.
2. Spread with margarine while hot to soften it further.
3. Add a thin layer of jelly, ensuring it contains no seeds or chunks.
4. Cut into small squares for easier chewing.

Adaptation notes: If unable to tolerate spreads, serve the toast plain or with margarine only. For allergies to grapes, use a permitted jelly in another flavor, provided it is smooth.

Snack: Vanilla Pudding Cup (Phase 1 and beyond)

Ingredients:

- 1 cup lactose-free milk or fortified almond/soy beverage (unsweetened)
- 2 tablespoons vanilla instant pudding mix

Instructions:

1. Whisk pudding mix and cold milk or beverage until thick, about 2 minutes.
2. Pour into a serving cup and chill until set, at least 30 minutes.
3. Stir before eating to ensure smoothness.

Adaptation notes: For dairy allergies, only use non-dairy beverages. Ensure the pudding mix is nut-free and does not include high-fiber additives.

Main: Broiled White Fish and Canned Green Beans (Phase 1 and Phase 2)

Ingredients:

- 4 oz boneless, skinless white fish fillet (such as cod or tilapia)
- 1 teaspoon olive oil or soft margarine
- Pinch of salt
- 1/2 cup canned green beans, drained

Instructions:

1. Preheat broiler.
2. Place fish fillet on a foil-lined tray, brush with oil or margarine.
3. Sprinkle salt, broil until opaque and flakes with a fork (8-10 minutes depending on thickness).
4. Warm green beans in a pan or microwave, steaming until very soft.
5. Plate fish and beans side by side; mash beans with a fork for easier swallowing.

Adaptation notes: For fish allergies, substitute with mashed hard-boiled eggs or soft tofu. For seasoning, add a squeeze of lemon if tolerated.

Snack: Gelatin with Applesauce (Phase 1 and Phase 2)

Ingredients:

- 1/2 cup prepared plain gelatin (avoid fruit chunks)
- 1/4 cup smooth applesauce

Instructions:

1. Chill gelatin until firm.
2. Spoon gelatin into a dish and top with applesauce.
3. Serve cold for a refreshing, easy-to-swallow snack.

Adaptation notes: Applesauce must not contain peel or chunks. Substitute with canned pears mashed smooth if the apple is not tolerated.

Side: Creamy Mashed Potatoes (Phase 1 and 2)

Ingredients:

- 1 medium white potato (peeled)
- 2 tablespoons lactose-free milk or broth
- 1 teaspoon margarine or butter
- Pinch of salt

Instructions:

1. Peel and cut potato into small pieces.
2. Boil until fully soft, about 15 minutes.
3. Drain and mash with milk and margarine until smooth and lump-free.
4. Add salt to taste and serve warm.

Adaptation notes: For milk allergies, use clear broth or water. Add more margarine for moisture if needed.

Ingredient Swap Sub-Guide: Allergies, Substitutions, and Budget Adjustments

Not all staples are suitable for every household or budget, and allergies can add another layer of complexity. Each core ingredient can be swapped to match health needs, local availability, or financial reality—here is a quick sub-guide:

- **Dairy:** Replace milk, yogurt, and cheese with lactose-free or fortified plant-based options (soy, oat, rice, almond). Use plain, unflavored varieties to avoid additives or fibers.
- **Protein:** Swap chicken for firm tofu or canned fish (packed in water, not oil) for cost-saving or meat-free diets. Always drain thoroughly and break into small, soft pieces. For eggs, use pasteurized liquid egg substitute for those allergic to whole eggs.
- **Grains:** If white bread or pasta is not available, use white corn grits, plain white bagels, or rice porridge—ensuring all are free of seeds, nuts, and whole grains.
- **Vegetables:** Use canned vegetables for convenience and economics, always choosing "no salt added" if possible, and avoid anything with visible skins, seeds, or stringy fibers.
- **Fruits:** Applesauce, mashed bananas, or canned peaches (peeled) can stand in for more expensive fruits; always buy unsweetened and check texture.
- **Fats:** Margarine, small amounts of vegetable oil, or plain butter are allowed; swap as needed for local and economic reasons.
- **Desserts:** Prepare plain cakes, cookies, and puddings at home with allowed flours and milks to lower costs and control texture.

- **Snacks:** White pretzels, simple vanilla wafers, and plain crackers substitute for branded or specialty items. Avoid whole grains, seeds, and popcorn.
- **Sauces:** Make plain gravy or broth at home from scraps to avoid commercial thickeners, seeds, and hidden fiber.
- **Cultural swaps:** White rice can be replaced by congee; potatoes by mashed, peeled yuca; and plain pasta by soft-cooked rice noodles, if appropriate and soft enough.

Always match the final dish's texture and moisture to low-fiber requirements, regardless of which ingredient list you use.

Stepwise Preparation Walkthroughs: Bringing Recipes to Life

Success with recipes hinges on careful preparation, especially with peeling, softening, and blending steps. The following tips are essential across all dishes:

- Use low, steady heat for boiling or steaming grains, vegetables, or proteins. Sudden high heat can toughen texture or brown surfaces, making foods harder to digest.
- Always peel fruits and vegetables. The skin harbors most of the fiber, even on canned or store-bought produce. Remove seeds entirely, even from soft produce.
- For proteins, use moist cooking methods: baking with foil, poaching in broth, steaming, or gently scrambling eggs. Hard searing leaves crusty edges best avoided.
- For grains, add extra water and cook until soft enough to mash with a fork.

- For snack and dessert assembly, chill finished gelatin or pudding fully before serving for a smoother mouthfeel and easier swallowing.
- If the result feels too dry, add a drizzle of safe fat or broth on top immediately before serving.
- Use foods from a single recipe in multiple forms. For example, leftover mashed potatoes can be thinned into a creamy soup with broth, or broiled fish can be mashed with rice for a light lunch.

Portioning and Presentation for Gentle Intake

Serving too much at once can trigger symptoms or leave you fearful of eating. Use a gentle presentation model:

- Serve smaller amounts one cup or less of any grain or vegetable side, and 2-3 ounces of protein per meal.
- Use small plates or bowls to make servings look substantial, which can help with appetite.
- Cut or mash all items before presenting, so no tough skin or large piece remains.
- Moisture matters: drizzle sauces or permitted fats over grains and proteins just before serving, preventing dryness.
- Allow food to cool slightly; heat increases scent and can cause nausea when appetite is low.
- Offer one or two colors per plate: for example, white rice, orange carrot, and pale chicken, or white bread, pale pink pudding, and yellow banana.
- If trying a new food, eat it by itself at first. Wait at least an hour before adding another new food. This helps spot any reaction or symptom.

Recipe Troubleshooting Guide: Spotting Intolerance and Adjusting on the Fly

Symptoms sometimes flare even when following all the rules. Clues that a meal is causing trouble include:

- Stomach pain or cramping within minutes or up to several hours after eating.
- Bloating or excessive fullness, especially after new components.
- Change in bowel movement consistency or urgency after specific meals.
- New food aversions, especially to textures previously well-tolerated.

When symptoms occur, adjust quickly:

- Switch back to softer, blander versions of the meal. For instance, if a whole cooked carrot causes gas, puree it next time or swap for canned green beans.
- Remove any item eaten for the first time in the most recent meal until symptoms settle.
- Return to proven "safe" items for the next few meals: tried-and-tested scrambled eggs, mashed potatoes, white rice, pudding.
- For any processed or canned item, check the ingredient list for hidden fiber, seeds, nuts, or unapproved vegetables; these can sometimes be introduced by changing brands or formulations.
- If symptoms continue for more than two days or get worse, stop all new ads and call your health care provider.

Keep a diary of what was eaten, how it was prepared, texture, and portion—this is your best tool for identifying patterns and avoiding repeated upsets.

The recipes and swaps provided here are both starting points and practical tools for managing your nutrition independently. By combining gentle cooking, careful portioning, and troubleshooting, you can respond quickly to the unpredictable realities of a sensitive digestive tract. Every household and individual will develop a unique routine, shaped by food access, specific tolerances, and evolving preferences.

As you practice these approaches, your confidence in selecting, preparing, and modifying recipes grows. Symptoms become manageable data points, not mysterious setbacks. Meals return to being moments of nourishment, comfort, and even pleasure, as you find new favorites and adapt old ones with skill and care. Always remain open to support from your health provider or nutritionist to ensure all nutrient needs are met for as long as a low fiber, low residue plan is needed.

Eating well on this plan is not about giving up flavor or joy. It's about learning flexible, solid fundamentals, smooth textures, careful swaps, gentle presentation, and rapid troubleshooting—so that you can approach your meals calmly, even on tough days.

Troubleshooting, Long-Term Adaptation, and Personalized Strategies

When eating on a low fiber, low residue plan, the hardest part is not just finding "safe" foods. The real test is staying comfortable as your body changes, keeping meals interesting, and speaking up when old patterns are challenged, especially in social or work settings. This chapter takes a hands-on look at what to do when things go wrong, how to break boredom, how to safely experiment, and what it means to keep your plan truly personal.

Let's move step by step through each challenge starting with real-world troubleshooting and ending with the tools you need for the future.

Digestive Symptom Troubleshooting: Step-by-Step Issue Fixing

When symptoms return or do not improve, clarity beats guessing. Using observations and simple records, you can untangle what is happening and take early action before small problems grow.

Start with symptoms: pain, bloating, constipation, nutrition shortfalls, or sudden changes after eating a new meal. **Here is a practical way to match a symptom to action.**

- **Stomach pain or cramping:** Ask yourself when the pain starts relative to meals. Pain right after eating a new food, or a new combination of foods, means the meal may be too hard to digest at your current stage. It can also mean the food, though technically "allowed," might still be too firm, rich, or irritating right now. Go back to softer foods—mashed potatoes, pudding, smooth eggs or plain white rice—and monitor closely.
- **Bloating and excess fullness:** Bloating, especially with cramping, often links to foods that ferment or remain in the gut too long. This can result from hidden fiber, unpeeled vegetables, or eating too fast. Also, be alert for dairy if you are lactose intolerant. Try reducing portion sizes, slowing down meals, favoring very soft textures, and, if using dairy, swap to lactose-free options or cut back for a few days. Track which meal combinations bring this on.
- **Constipation, or bowel "slowdown":** The diet naturally cuts bulk-forming fiber, which can slow the bowels. However, sharp drops in meal size, dehydration, or extended reliance on very refined foods without enough fluid can worsen this. Add extra fluids like clear juice, water, or strained vegetable broth. Use approved, moist fruits like bananas or smooth applesauce. Review your day's menu—are you only eating bread, crackers, and protein? Work in cooked vegetables and canned fruit from the approved list.

- **Diarrhea or loose stools:** For some, even a low residue plan can spark diarrhea, especially if dairy, sweeteners, or high-fat foods are increased. Diarrhea accompanied by urgency, cramping, or repeated returns to the bathroom after new foods likely signals intolerance or a new trigger. Revert to a "safer" day of known foods, such as plain white bread, white rice, soft eggs, and dairy alternatives if needed. Cut out foods newly tried in the past 24 hours.
- **Signs of nutrition shortfall:** Fast weight loss, rising fatigue, or picky eating can creep up on this restrictive plan. Warning signs include skipping entire meal groups (such as avoiding protein or all fruit), persistent weakness, or needing to rest after simple activities. If you hit the two-week mark on the diet, or cut entire food groups, take a multivitamin with minerals and reach out to your doctor or a dietitian for review.

If any symptom persists beyond three days, or you notice blood in stool, unrelenting vomiting, black stools, fevers, severe dehydration, or pain that does not ease, escalate promptly to your health provider.

Keeping Meals Engaging: Breaking Monotony, Sparking Enjoyment

The plan can quickly lose its appeal if every dish tastes the same or you feel cornered by bland foods. The key to sticking with this approach is to rotate flavors, textures, and presentation styles. Try these methods to add variety without breaking the plan's core boundaries.

- **Rotate protein sources:** Even if you stick to tender, well-cooked options, swap between chicken, broiled lean beef, poached fish, and eggs through the week. Use canned tuna or jack mackerel, mashed and seasoned simply, to bring in new taste.
- **Change preparation, not the ingredient:** Baked chicken one day, gently scrambled eggs the next, followed by soft poached fish, all work differently on the palate and the mood.
- **Add allowed sauces and flavorings:** Spoon a little butter, olive oil, or mayonnaise over meats and rice. Use smooth salad dressing, clear jelly, honey, or syrup on white bread or pudding. Soy sauce and strained dressings help keep themes from repeating daily.
- **Use broth to soften:** Cooking grains or pasta with plain broth (or vegetables in a mild chicken stock) gives flavor depth without extra fiber. Serve rice or pasta as a "side soup" sometimes, with more liquid, for day-to-day change.
- **Play with temperature:** Serve some foods chilled (gelatin, puddings, applesauce), others warm (mashed potatoes, softly steamed vegetables, risottos). Texture and scent shift with temperature and comfort level.
- **Build plates with color:** Even within the brief "allowed" list, alternate orange from carrots, yellow from potatoes or butter, green from well-cooked beans or soft lettuce, and white from bread or eggs.
- **Use fruit for contrast:** Soft banana slices on a plate with bread, chilled applesauce as a side, or drained canned peaches with dinner.

- **Keep a food and symptom diary:** Note which combinations feel tiring or spark cravings for missed flavors. Rotate foods out before you tire of them completely, cycling back to favorites after breaks.

Pacing and Setbacks: Approaching Reintroduction Safely

After acute symptoms ease, the urge to bring back fruits, vegetables, and whole grains grows. Safe reintroduction is not about a single decision. Instead, take a staged route so you can spot setbacks quickly and prevent a cycle of flare-ups and restrictions.

Start only after three straight days of mild or no symptoms. Pick one new food—cooked, peeled, and portioned small. For instance, add half a peeled, cooked carrot or a quarter cup of canned pears. Eat it separately, not mixed into larger dishes, and monitor for 24–48 hours. If no increased pain, bloating, or changes in bowel patterns, add another new item, following the same process.

Return to your basic plan if symptoms return. Do not introduce multiple new foods at once. Step back to tolerated, proven options—mashed potatoes, soft-cooked rice, plain eggs or tofu—for at least two "safe" meals before trying again.

Take special care with foods high in lactose, roughage, or seeds. For dairy, always use lactose-free if you ever experienced cramping or loose stools after milk. Try dairy items in smaller servings at first (half a cup or less) and pause before moving up.

If you must remain on this diet for over two weeks due to a slow recovery or repeated setbacks, supplement with a multivitamin/mineral once daily, and work with a doctor or registered nutritionist to avoid slow nutritional decline. If a setback includes weight loss, persistent fatigue, or loss of appetite, escalate more quickly.

Communicating Needs in Social, Medical, and Work Settings

Navigating meals in group settings is often more stressful than sticking to the menu at home. Peer pressure, misunderstandings, and lack of awareness can put you in awkward spots. Being prepared with a simple explanation saves energy and conflict.

Strategies to speak up clearly:

- **For friends or family gatherings:** "I'm following a temporary medical diet that means I need soft, low-fiber foods for a few weeks. Would it be okay if I bring my own meal, or can I help plan a menu with you?"
- **For work meals or eating out:** "For health reasons, I need simple foods without raw vegetables or whole grains just for now. I'll check the menu for options like plain meats, white bread, and soft-cooked foods."
- **For clinicians, nurses, or hospital staff:** "I am on a medically-advised low fiber, low residue diet due to [diagnosis]. Here's a list of foods I can and cannot eat, provided by my health provider. Could you help make sure any meals fit this plan?"

Prepare a one-page food list to hand over, listing allowed and not allowed foods, based on your stage. Keep this in your phone, on a notepad, or as a small printed card. If plans change or menu options are limited, suggest suitable alternatives or request a plain item from the kitchen, such as soft rice or eggs. Any time a host or staff member is uncertain, politely offer to review options together.

When advocating for your diet, keep your tone neutral and fact-based. Most people are willing to help once they understand restrictions are temporary and supported by your health provider. If met with resistance, reiterate your medical need and, if in a healthcare setting, ask for dietary services to help ensure your needs are respected.

Personalized Recovery Plan: Building a Flexible Roadmap

Diet adaptation only works if built around your actual needs, day-to-day life, and body signals. Use this worksheet-style guide to shape your next steps, spot trouble, and stay on track even as healing progresses.

1. **Track baseline**: For the next four days, write down each meal and snack, noting portion sizes, preparation, and how you felt 1 and 24 hours after eating. Write down bowel patterns and any discomfort.
2. **Set short-term goals: These might be:**

   o Two days in a row without pain or cramping,

   o Eating three balanced meals daily using soft, approved foods,

- o Gradually reintroducing one new food every 48 hours after 3 symptom-free days,
- o Keeping hydration up, aiming for at least six glasses of liquid per day.

3. **Define your "safe list":** List all foods and preparations consistently tolerated in the past week. This includes plain bread, white rice, mashed potatoes, eggs, certain canned fruits, and safe beverages. These are your fallback items for flare days.
4. **Map warning signs that require escalation:** If any of these occur, halt new food testing and contact your care provider if:
   - o Pain does not ease after two days of strict low residue eating,
   - o Bowel habits change suddenly to blood, black, or tarry stool,
   - o Recurrent vomiting, severe constipation or diarrhea lasting more than 48 hours,
   - o Loss of appetite for three days, or sudden weight drop.
5. **Plan rotations:** Make a weekly rotation plan using at least two proteins, three permitted sides, and various fruit options. Cycle through sauces and cooking styles, noting any dips in appetite or enjoyment to adjust rotation.
6. **Recheck nutrition:** Each week, review if every core group protein, grains, fruit/vegetable, permitted fat is represented. Adjust with allowable alternatives or ask for help from nutrition services if groups are missed repeatedly.
7. **Maintenance:** Once in a stable phase (no new symptoms for one week), transition to testing new foods, always following the single change at a time pace, and returning to your safe list at the first sign of upset.

This worksheet becomes a living plan growing as you learn what works, helping your support team revisit and adjust your diet, and acting as your safety net during future flares or medical procedures.

Adapting to a low fiber, low residue plan is more than restricting foods for a few days or weeks. It is a test of attention: to the signals from your body, the triggers in your surroundings, and the changing patterns in your social and family life.

Commit to troubleshooting each symptom with a record and response mindset. Refresh your menu often and make use of the many allowed combinations of simple, gently prepared foods—no single option needs to be eaten more than three days in a row if planning ahead with swaps and rotations. Pace yourself when reintroducing new options. Resist pressure to rush, and step back promptly at the first trouble sign.

Speak up at every table, whether at home, the workplace, a cafeteria, or hospital, and carry your needs with assurance. Most setbacks are temporary if met early, with disciplined troubleshooting and clear meal planning based on your own clear feedback.

Regularly update your written plan and consult your support system, especially after weeks of restriction, unusual symptoms, or eroding appetite. Add a multivitamin with minerals when the diet extends, and do not hesitate to check in with a doctor or trained nutritionist. Consistency builds skill, and variety however small keeps you motivated to stick with recovery, grow your options, and rebuild not just your gut health but your enjoyment of food itself.

Conclusion

A successful journey with a low fiber low residue diet depends on understanding the purpose and strengths of its structured approach. This guide's 2-phase plan beginning with strict restriction for flare management and progressing to gradual reintroduction during recovery provides a practical framework for restoring comfort and stability in digestive health. By following the detailed food lists, meal plans, and recipes, individuals are empowered to make informed choices and confidently navigate fluctuating symptoms while minimizing dietary guesswork.

The two-phase system offers clear benefits: Phase 1 creates an environment of digestive rest, reducing physical irritation for those experiencing acute symptoms from conditions such as IBD flares or post-operative healing. This period of dietary simplicity often brings rapid relief, decreased stool output, and eased abdominal discomfort. Phase 2, with its carefully calibrated reintroduction of foods, allows the gut to gradually regain tolerance and nutritional diversity while monitoring for recurrence of issues. This stepwise process supports sustained recovery, promoting safe expansion of the diet without abrupt setbacks.

An essential part of success with this diet is ongoing symptom monitoring and the flexibility to individualize adjustments. Keeping a daily log of meals and symptoms helps you spot patterns and quickly identify foods that do not agree with your system. Tracking weight, energy levels, and gastrointestinal changes makes it easier to catch nutritional gaps or complications early.

Since everyone's digestive response and nutritional needs are unique, this individualized feedback coupled with input from your healthcare provider or dietitian ensures that you remain in control and adaptive, rather than rigidly following a static list.

For long-term gut health maintenance, the next steps emphasize gradual transition, balanced nutrition, and proactive communication. As your condition stabilizes, work with your medical team to tailor reintroduction speed and select foods that maximize both satisfaction and nutritional adequacy.

Don't rush to abandon all restrictions; some individuals will discover personal trigger foods that remain problematic well into remission or recovery. The skills gained by reading labels, experimenting with new recipes, and advocating for your needs in social settings will remain valuable beyond the acute phase.

Continuing to prioritize gut health involves more than dietary vigilance. Emphasize adequate hydration, consider supplemental vitamins or minerals if advised, and schedule regular medical follow-ups to track progress. Cultivate flexibility in meal planning so that your approach can ebb and flow with your unique symptoms, lifestyle, and preferences. Remember: The value of a low fiber low residue diet is not just in short-term relief, but in the knowledge and resilience you build to support your digestive health now and in the future.

FAQs

What is the difference between a low-fiber and low-residue diet, and which one should I follow?

A low-fiber diet restricts plant fiber, like tough vegetable skins, whole grains, and raw fruits, to limit undigested roughage. A low-residue diet goes further: it cuts out fiber and also restricts foods that increase bowel residue in other ways such as beans, some dairy (limited to 2 cups/day), and tougher meats. Thus, a low-residue diet is more restrictive.

Your provider will specify the right approach for your needs, especially for post-surgical recovery, flares, or risk of obstruction. When in doubt, check with your provider.

See Chapter 1 for a deeper explanation of fiber, residue, and digestive function.

Which foods are allowed and which must be avoided?

The foundation of this diet is knowing your safe and restricted foods. Approved options include:

- White bread, rolls, and baked goods with refined white flour only (no bran, seeds, or whole grains)
- White rice, plain pasta, peeled potatoes
- Cooked or canned fruits/vegetables without skins or seeds (applesauce, strained juices, ripe bananas, cooked pumpkin)

- Lean, tender meats and eggs
- Milk and dairy within the limit (max 2 cups per day), if tolerated
- Juices and beverages with no pulp or seeds

Avoid whole grains, nuts, seeds, dried or raw fruits, tough/fatty meats, beans, fruit/veg skins, and high-fat foods. Some fiber-free foods are restricted if they increase bowel residue. For more detailed, adaptive lists (vegetarian, lactose-free, etc.), see Chapter 4.

Can I meet my nutrient needs on this diet, and how do I avoid deficiencies?

These diets limit many foods rich in essential nutrients. Over time (especially after two weeks), you risk deficiency in vitamins A, C, K, B6, folate, and minerals like magnesium and potassium, as well as dietary fiber.

If following this diet for more than two weeks, take a daily multivitamin with minerals. If you notice fatigue, poor healing, or hair loss, consult your provider.

For more on deficiency risks, monitoring, and supplements, see Chapter 5.

How do I manage eating out, travel, or social events with these restrictions?

Success in real-world situations depends on planning, communicating assertively, and having emergency safe foods ready.

- Travel: Bring shelf-stable approved foods (plain crackers, applesauce, canned fruits). Identify grocery stores or restaurants offering safe basics—white bread, eggs, plain soups.

- Social events: Let hosts know your restrictions, offer to bring a permitted dish, and watch for hidden ingredients like grains or seeds.
- Dining out: Opt for venues providing simple items (baked chicken, mashed potatoes without skin, canned fruit). Ask about ingredients and request substitutions.

Comorbidities like lactose intolerance or diabetes require extra care—seek lactose-free dairy or lactase supplements as needed. For adaptive strategies, see Chapter 7 and Chapter 8.

Are there special guidelines for lactose intolerance, diabetes, or other dietary restrictions?

Yes, special dietary needs must be incorporated. For lactose intolerance, keep dairy under two cups daily or use lactose-free or suitable plant alternatives. If diabetic, note that permitted foods like white bread and rice spike glucose quickly; pair with protein, space meals, and monitor blood sugar.

Anyone with allergies or complex medical conditions should adjust the plan with a registered dietitian. More help for mixed dietary needs is in Chapters 4 and 7.

When and how do I stop the diet or reintroduce foods?

These diets are temporary, aiming to control symptoms and support healing. Transitioning off should be gradual unless otherwise directed. Expansion begins when symptoms improve (less pain, normalized bowel habits) and your provider gives clearance.

When reintroducing, slowly increase daily fiber, add back one new group at a time, and monitor for symptoms. Hydrate well during this period. For stepwise guides, see Chapter 3 and Chapter 9.

What warning signs mean I should contact my provider immediately?

Seek immediate advice for:

- Persistent pain, vomiting, or abdominal distension despite following the diet
- Signs of deficiency: major fatigue, new hair loss, slow healing, frequent infections
- Difficulty maintaining weight or signs of dehydration (dark urine, dizziness)
- Ongoing diarrhea, constipation, or any blood in stool

For more on escalation and troubleshooting, see Chapters 2 and 9.

References and Helpful Links

Spiller, G., Amen, R., Kritchevsky, D.. (1975). Dietary fiber in human nutrition. *C R C Critical Reviews in Food Science and Nutrition.* https://doi.org/10.1080/10408397509527201

Liu, M., Zhou, S., Li, Y. et al.. (2021). Structure, physicochemical properties and effects on nutrients digestion of modified soluble dietary fiber extracted from sweet potato residue. *Food Research International.* https://doi.org/10.1016/j.foodres.2021.110761

Putri, R., Amalia, F., Utami, F. et al.. (2025). One-day low-residue diet is equally effective as the multiple-day low-residue diet in achieving adequate bowel cleansing: a meta-analysis of randomized controlled trials. *Clinical Endoscopy.* https://doi.org/10.5946/ce.2024.061

Layman, D.. (1986). Nutrition and Exercise: An Overview. *ACS Symposium Series.* https://doi.org/10.1021/bk-1986-0294.ch001

Vanhauwaert, E., Matthys, C., Verdonck, L. et al.. (2015). Low-Residue and Low-Fiber Diets in Gastrointestinal Disease Management. *Advances in Nutrition.* https://doi.org/10.3945/an.115.009688

Unknown Author. (2019). Dietary Interventions in Gastrointestinal Diseases. Elsevier. https://doi.org/10.1016/c2017-0-01390-3

Rossi, R., Whyand, T., Murray, C. et al.. (2016). The role of dietary supplements in inflammatory bowel disease: a systematic review. *European Journal of Gastroenterology & Hepatology.* https://doi.org/10.1097/meg.0000000000000728

Jofré, A., Latorre-Moratalla, M., Garriga, M. et al.. (2019). Domestic refrigerator temperatures in Spain: Assessment of its impact on the safety and shelf-life of cooked meat products. *Food Research International.* https://doi.org/10.1016/j.foodres.2019.108578

Taylor, S., Baumert, J.. (2010). Cross-Contamination of Foods and Implications for Food Allergic Patients. *Current Allergy and Asthma Reports*. https://doi.org/10.1007/s11882-010-0112-4

Chen, H., Cheng, H., Wu, W. et al.. (2008). Supplementation of Konjac Glucomannan into a Low-Fiber Chinese Diet Promoted Bowel Movement and Improved Colonic Ecology in Constipated Adults: A Placebo-Controlled, Diet-Controlled Trial. *Journal of the American College of Nutrition*. https://doi.org/10.1080/07315724.2008.10719681

www.ingramcontent.com/pod-product-compliance
Lightning Source LLC
LaVergne TN
LVHW022008200926
848481LV00007B/2279